A Most Meaningful Life
my dad and Alzheimer's

The Comfort in their Journey Series
by Trish Laub

A Most Meaningful Life
my dad and Alzheimer's
a guide to living with dementia

Peaceful Endings
guiding the walk to the end of life and beyond
steps to take before and after

Through the Rabbit Hole
navigating the maze of providing care
a quick guide to care options and decisions

A Most Meaningful Life
my dad and Alzheimer's

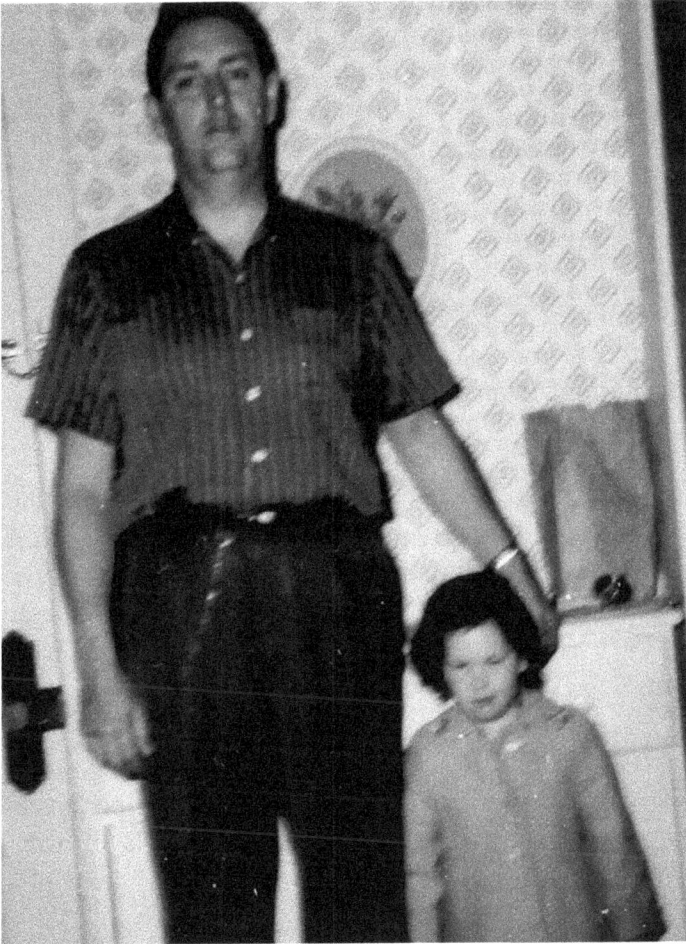

a guide to living with dementia

Trish Laub

PSM Publishing

A Most Meaningful Life, my dad and Alzheimer's
by Trish Laub

Author photo by Joanne Wagner
Published by PSM Publishing

ISBN-13: 978-1-7322006-0-9
Library of Congress Control Number: 2018939960
First Edition   Printed in the United States of America

PSM
ublishing

To purchase:
www.TrishLaub.com   720-288-0772
6845 Osprey Ct Highlands Ranch CO
80130

Dedication

To my dad

Everything that I am, I see in your eyes ...
always and forever.

vi

ACKNOWLEDGEMENTS

with special thanks to both Mom and Dad,

my husband, Chris, who supported my absence during this experience as well as the creation of this project,

my sisters, Barbara and Nancy, who lived my experience with me yet have their own experiences and stories to share,

my daughter Justine, who is my inspiration for all things,

the friends (Janice, Karen, Skye, Julia, Mia, Teilene and others) who have carried me through the dark times,

those who have encouraged me to shine a light down the path for those who come next,

Roseanne Geisel (editor), Joanne Wagner (author photographer), Krista Lee (logo and graphic designer), and Sophia Taylor (website/branding) all of whose excellence is unsurpassed,

Deb Sheppard, medium and mentor, who helped me with the "Great Clearing," making this project possible,

all of the caregivers who loved my parents and taught me so much: Margery, *Debbie, Lucia, Ann, Ruth, Shawn, David* and *Angel,* as well as many others who provided not only care but unconditionally gave love; they are all extraordinary people and I am proud to know them and to call them family,

and especially, *Margery, the caregiver* who encouraged me to write this book, which resulted in *Comfort in Their Journey* and the book series.

and finally a very special thank you to all those who agreed to be what I call my "small book" readers, those who read and provided invaluable feedback on the content: *Justine, Janice, Karen, Skye, Cathe, Margery, Ellen, Judy, Elisabeth, Susie, Klaralee, Debbie and Chris.*

CONTENTS

Chapter 10
UNDERSTANDING A LIFE WITH ALZHEIMER'S ...

Chapter 11
MY FAMILY'S STRATEGY ...

Chapter 12
HIS LEGACY ...

NOTES TO THE READER

Citation of Information
This book presents a conceptual understanding of information, terms, and statistics intended to assist you in a conversation with, and in asking questions of, a professional. Information, unless specifically cited, was provided to me during conversations with professionals or through research of many reliable sources. I have tried to simplify it for non-professionals.

Patient Advocacy
Patient advocacy is **the most important role** in regard to caring for another, and can literally be the difference between life and death. The topic is mentioned in every book of the Comfort in Their Journey book series. It is discussed in Chapters 6 and 11 of *A Most Meaningful Life* and Chapter 1 of *Peaceful Endings*. However, if you only read one chapter in the entire series, please read **The Need for Patient Advocacy... the most important role,** Chapter 2 in *"Through The Rabbit Hole."*

Pronouns
At some point in your life, it is almost certain that you will be responsible for the care of another person. It may be a parent, a sibling, a child or a friend. It may be a loved one, and it may be someone for whom you do not feel love. The gender and age will vary. These variables make it difficult when writing a book and having to reference the person for whom you are responsible for providing care. Therefore, in this text, in regard to the gender, the pronoun "their," as a genderless person, may be used.

About the Ladybugs

The ladybug has been an obsession for me since I was very young and began to collect them. My dad named his fishing boats Ladybug and Ladybug II. The use of the ladybug is an homage to my dad, and the red color, my mom's favorite and her most recent nail color, an homage to her.

Comfort in their J🐞urney
with *Trish Laub*

You may notice that the *Comfort in Their Journey* logo incorporates the ladybug as the "o" in the word journey.

The open-winged ladybug appears at the top of special sections, such as the Dedication and the start of the Contents, and on the page prior to the start of each chapter.

The closed-winged ladybug appears at the start of each subchapter. In addition, while all information in the book is important, the presence of 🐞🐞 two closed-winged ladybugs is used to indicate information that requires additional attention. The presence of 🐞🐞🐞 three closed-winged ladybugs indicates especially critical information.

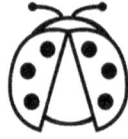

Knowledge is Power.
Francis Bacon

PREFACE ...
an unlikely expert ...
and "short is the new black"

I became an unlikely "expert"; it's as simple as that. I am not a medical, legal or financial professional. My expertise is derived from the full-time care of my parents, one with Alzheimer's, for whom I delivered the total care and the end-of-life experience that my parents desired.

In the book "Outliers," the author Malcolm Gladwell speaks to what truly makes someone reach their potential for success. He shares that more than IQ, and in addition to many other factors, practice is key to becoming successful. The principle states that 10,000 hours of "practice" or experience that pushes the skill set to the brink are needed to achieve mastery in any field.

Recently there was an ad for Denver's UCHealth in which Peyton Manning says: "It takes 10,000 hours to become an expert at something. But what happens at 20,000 hours? Or 30,000 hours? What happens when you dedicate yourself to it? Do you become something greater? A leader? A mentor? An innovator? At a certain point, it seems, you stop playing the game and start changing it."

My experience puts me well over 12,000 hours of "practice." Does it make me an expert? Maybe, but only on what I experienced. And after experiencing what I have, it might have seemed "easy" to just walk away and never talk about it or share what I have learned with anyone. To simply "move on." But, I couldn't do it -- walk away with all that I have learned and experienced. It became a "calling," the desire to share in hopes that it might help even one other person thrive in a situation which many times offers only frustration and often defeat. A calling, but was I an expert? Yes, and I am qualified.

What am I qualified to offer? I offer my story and my experience. It is highly likely that during your lifetime you will be responsible for the care of a person with a severe health issue and equally as likely that it will be during the final years and days of that person's life. I offer you the opportunity to *thrive* throughout the process, to think and then take action.

I am here to offer you information, some direction and suggested questions to ask.
- I am not a medical professional; I am not providing medical advice.
- I am not a legal professional; I am not providing legal advice.
- I am not a financial professional; I am not providing financial advice.

During my experience, I needed information I didn't know how to find, and I needed it quickly. Since my experience, I have found that there are hundreds of books and organizations offering pieces of the information I needed. And while the Internet offers information, extreme caution and verification are necessary to ensure accurate and useful advice. In many cases I didn't even know where to look for it or the terminology to Google or to ask. In other cases, I had too little time to find, read and understand it all. I needed the Reader's Digest version of everything. I needed a guide: a clear, concise and useable quick reference. With that in mind, I have adopted the philosophy that "short is the new black" – it is not the volume of words but the value of them that is useful; that providing you with lists and bullet points, things to consider, questions to ask and leads to follow are the most helpful delivery of information.

I also want to state up front that many factors, ranging from geographic proximity to financial resources to flexibility of work schedules, determine what is possible for every family or caregiving team. Each family or caregiving team will handle things in a way suitable for them and the person relying on them. My hope is to provide you tips and spark ideas that work for you.

In short, I became an unlikely expert; I have lived what I have to share.

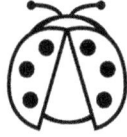

Every 67 seconds
someone is diagnosed with Alzheimer's.
The Alzheimer's Association

PROLOGUE ...
Alzheimer's,
the tip of an epidemic of dementia

Until recently Alzheimer's has been shrouded in secrecy and shame, as though those diagnosed with it had anything to do with having it. It was a confusing, dark and depressing diagnosis, served with the frightening knowledge that it is not curable. People didn't talk about it when Alzheimer's hit their families. They whispered about it because of the stigma attached to the disease. There was little information and even less hope. It was thought to be "an old person's disease" from which they would eventually die.

Today, every 67 seconds someone is diagnosed with Alzheimer's. We are literally headed toward a national emergency. According to the Alzheimer's Association, by the year 2050 there will be a projected 16 million people diagnosed with Alzheimer's in the United States, requiring an estimated 80 million caregivers, and costing a staggering $1.1 trillion for care. Globally that number is stunning: 160 million diagnosed requiring 800 million caregivers and costing an unimaginable amount.

Dementia is the umbrella under which Alzheimer's falls. The Alzheimer's Association says that approximately 1 in 7, 13.9% of Americans age 71 or older will have some type of dementia. 70% of those with dementia will have Alzheimer's. With the aging of the Baby Boomers, projections are increasing steadily. Clearly, Alzheimer's is the tip of an epidemic.

We need to talk about Alzheimer's. Nationally, locally, with friends, with family, with anyone who will listen, and with those who don't want to listen. That is what I want to do here…. to talk about my experience with Alzheimer's in hopes that it helps even only one of you.

Alzheimer's is not a single disease entity, but rather a spectrum disorder that presents with different symptoms, progresses differently, and responds differently to treatment, with different prognoses, for each person.
Gayatri Devi from *The Spectrum of Hope*

I want to be clear, that as a doctor once said to Maria Shriver, "Once you've seen one case of Alzheimer's, you've seen…one case of Alzheimer's." This seems to be a disease that plays out differently for nearly every patient.

The Alzheimer's Association says, "There is no cure, prevention or treatment to slow the progression." However, there are effective medications, the symptoms and side effects of the disease are treatable and quality of life is possible. There are also new advances in the treatment. My story is exactly that. It is my story, my experience with my dad, and it is one of limitless possibilities.

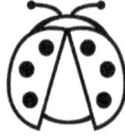

His life intersected with,
and profoundly changed,
mine.
Margery

INTRODUCTION ....
a most meaningful life to the end

MEMORIES OF FRANK
By a caregiver

Starting a new caregiving job is always a bit overwhelming – there is so much to learn so fast. In the case of Frank's family, this was especially true. I had to find my way around the kitchen, learn where everything was, find out where the supplies were kept, the linens, etc. There was the pill routine for Frank and the feeding routine. All pills crushed, and all food pureed to prevent swallowing mishaps. Jean's food and the food for the rest of the family had to be prepared separately, although we tried to use that food for Frank as well. Then there was learning the names of all the other caregivers. Debbie, the woman who trained me, said: "This is the easiest job you will ever have." I didn't believe her for a minute!

Everyone congregated in the small room off the kitchen – the sitting room. With separate caregivers for Frank and Jean, that little room was the center of much activity and action. Frank had his recliner in the center of the room, and Jean sat off on the far side of the room in her chair. The caregivers sat either in one of the remaining chairs, or on one of the barstools at the bar, which was open to the kitchen. As I said, it was a crowded room, with both people and activity.

When I started working for Frank, I felt like I had a terrible secret that I had to keep from the family. I wasn't sure if I could care for a man. I had mixed feelings about men, especially older men. My own father had been abusive. I carried this secret and unspoken baggage into the job with

5

Frank. I was wary of him at first. I'm not sure exactly when that changed. I think it was when he started calling me "Mommy." He called all his female caregivers "Mommy." It was too much for him to remember our names, so we were simply all "Mommy." I had the special privilege of being called, "Pretty Mommy."

Well, my heart began to melt. I started to realize that Frank was different from my cold and aloof and scary dad. And Frank was vulnerable – he needed care. And I was there to give him that care. I learned to put my feelings aside with the urgent necessity of providing that care for him. I think when I finally realized that, unlike my own father, Frank could not hurt me, and, in fact, didn't want to hurt me, I began to finally just do my job.

It didn't take long for Frank to win me over. He was just so… nice. That was out of context for me. None of the men in my life had been nice. This was something different. I started to feel a new affection for Frank, and I started looking forward to coming to work for him. I mastered the complicated routines of the job: the pills, the cooking, the pureeing of food, the interactions with the other caregivers, etc.

There were two experiences that I treasured while working for Frank. One was seeing his reaction when Jean entered the sitting room. He would look first, then recognize her, then say, "MOMMY," and his face would light up with pure delight. He was like a love-struck teenager when Jean came into the room. Not even his advanced illness could dim his love and recognition for his beloved. That special bond brought happiness into my heart. He was always just so happy to see her.

The other thing that I treasured was just watching the special relationship that Frank had with each of his daughters. There was enjoyment and playfulness there. I never tired of watching these interactions. Each of the three daughters had a distinctly different relationship with their father. Barb, the eldest daughter, was always friendly with him, but more polite and formal than the younger two daughters. She would come into the room and say, "Hi, dad," and she would just be there with him. There was a comfortableness about her relationship with Frank. He clearly enjoyed having her there.

With Nancy, who I always thought was the most like her dad, there was always the joking and playful quality. Nancy could get Frank to do anything that we were having trouble doing, like going down the hall to the bathroom. "Come on, dad," she would say. "I'll race you!" She had a very special way of joking with her father and getting him to laugh and smile. She met Frank right where he was, and everything was OK. I always felt comfortable with Nancy and enjoyed the fact that Frank was always so happy to see her.

Trish, the youngest daughter, was just that – the youngest, and she enjoyed the special relationship with her father that the youngest sometimes has. I remember her just coming in, always barefoot, and sitting down at her father's feet, and talking to him. Again, like Nancy, she met Frank right where he was. She was the practical daughter, always with a new project to make Frank more comfortable, like teaching us how to do the special treatments with the copper rods and plates. She was the practical daughter, mercurial in a way, and in some ways the favorite. Like my younger sister had been in my family. Since Trish had hired me, I felt the most comfortable with her. She was my point of contact with the whole family.

There was always so much activity in that little room. There was drama. Frank started having his seizures, which scared everyone, and Jean had her medical crises. Both of them had unexpected trips to the hospital. There was worry. And most of all, there was caring for both of them. We, the caregivers, became like the extended family, drawn into the drama by our own sense of responsibility for both parents. We couldn't help but care. It was such a nice family. For me, with my background, it was especially meaningful, and pleasantly unfamiliar territory. I was just soaking up the experience every day that I was there.

When I left the employment there, mostly because I hurt my back at home and couldn't continue the level of care that Frank and Jean needed, I maintained contact with the family through Jean, with whom I started to work on a memory book. Each time I arrived at the condo to work on the memory book with Jean, it was like coming home in a way. I was delighted when the rest of the family became involved in the project, and we managed to finish it by Christmastime.

One day, I talked to Trish on the phone, and she told me that Frank was "transitioning." We would miss our coffee date. When, a couple of days later, my cell phone rang and I recognized Trish's number, I realized before I answered that Frank was gone. Trish confirmed it. I was sad.

In retrospect, you can never convince me that life doesn't have meaning, even in its final stages. As sick as Frank was when I came into the household, his life intersected with, and profoundly changed mine. Frank had a profound influence on me, personally. He taught me, among other things, not to be afraid of men. That was a huge lesson for me, one that I so badly needed to learn.

Frank had, even at the very end, **a most meaningful life**.

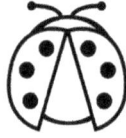

I cannot teach anybody anything,
I can only make them think.
Socrates

Chapter 1

IF IT WAS POSSIBLE FOR MY DAD ....
then it's possible

I have a story to share. I am a daughter who took the walk through Alzheimer's with my dad, a journey that did not come with a roadmap.

I cannot speak to what anyone else's experience with the disease will be. But after 12 years of treatment, and likely more living with Alzheimer's, the day on which my dad was last conscious he called me by name and spoke words of meaning only to me. He sat with my mom, held her hand, knew exactly who she was, and told her how much he loved her and that she was the love of his life. He was tired of living in the body that had carried him for 92 years, and it was time for him to go. That to me was the ultimate success!

Now consider this. Gunder Hagg, of Sweden, set the world record for running a mile in 4 minutes and 1.3 seconds in 1945. Athletes tried and failed, for many years, to run the mile in less than four minutes. It was, therefore, considered impossible. On May 6, 1954, Roger Bannister, became the first person to break that barrier coming in at 3 minutes 59.4 seconds. Interestingly, his world record in the mile run did not stand long, broken little more than one month later. Once broken, several factors such as improved surface conditions, and training and running techniques, contributed to the continual lowering of the record.

The point is that until the first person broke the record, it was thought to be impossible. I believe that if my dad and I could have the experience that we did, then it is possible for others too. My story is a success story, one of possibility and meaning. If it can happen for me, it is possible for you.

Through the story of our journey, I hope to inspire you to think, to know that even with Alzheimer's Disease the possibilities are limitless. With a clear philosophy and the creation of a strategy, you too can have a roadmap and navigate your loved one's journey so that they have "a most meaningful life."

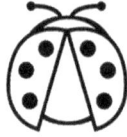

Being someone's first love may be great,
but to be their last is beyond perfect.
Unknown

Chapter 2

THE STARS OF THE STORY ...

a gentleman and his lady

While this story is primarily about my dad, it cannot be told without my mom.

My dad was a great man. He was a Denver native, attended North High School and the University of Denver. While in college, he was recruited for the Manhattan Project, government research that led to the atomic bomb. He declined that opportunity in order to enlist in the Navy during WWII. After his honorable discharge from the Navy, he was offered a top position with Sony in the development of the television tube but chose to join the FBI. While at the FBI he was offered a position with the first forensic lab. Dad ultimately spent most of his professional life as a salesman for Sanford Ink and was involved in the development of products including the Sharpie, Scented Mr. Sketch markers (that we called Smelly Markers), and Accent highlighters. He was inducted into the University of Denver's Hall of Fame for both Tennis and Basketball; played championship level tennis; and fished for over 80 years, which included being a Charter Boat Captain on Lake Michigan. To say that he was intelligent, accomplished and capable is an understatement.

My mom was the love of his life, and he hers. My mom was also a Denver native, attended East High School and the University of Denver where they met. She worked in a war plant during WWII and married my dad while he was on leave. She was a stay-at-home mom with three little girls but somehow managed to run a successful in-home international business selling quilted pillow kits, which were featured in magazines including Better Homes and Gardens and House Beautiful. She was at a minimum his equal.

Both were truly loving and kind.

My mom and dad were married for 69 years, and she was his anchor to reality, without which we could not have achieved success.

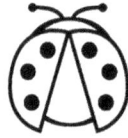

Life is 10% what happens to you
and
90% how you choose to respond to it.
Unknown

Chapter 3

DAD HAS ALZHEIMER'S ...
welcome to the new normal

My mom and dad were in town visiting for Christmas. They were on their way to my house after staying with my sister. I received a phone call from my sister with the news that our dad was being treated for Alzheimer's. I think for a moment my heart stopped, and I was devastated.

Soon after my dad was "diagnosed" with Alzheimer's, Maria Shriver's father was diagnosed. In an interview, she said that her husband gave her the best advice: to stop expecting her father to be who he had been before. In short, she needed to accept her father as who he is at the time, just as she would have if he were not living with Alzheimer's. The advice that Maria shared saved me!

My immediate concerns were that my dad would know that he had Alzheimer's, and that at some point he would suffer in some way. At that moment, I committed to doing everything in my power to see that it was going to have the smallest-possible negative impact on his life, and that he would not "suffer" a single moment.

And, I had great clarity that my dad was still my dad, nothing less. He most certainly was not the disease, and I would meet him wherever he was. My goal was to keep his life as normal as possible and as close as possible to the way he would have lived without Alzheimer's.

> Grief is the price of love,
> not a sign of weakness.
> Trish Laub

Then the emotions arrived in full force: shock, anger, fear, sadness and ultimately grief. I had always heard that Alzheimer's was a death sentence and briefly that thought consumed me. And then, in a moment I had a realization that shifted things for me. My dad could possibly die of something other than Alzheimer's! Yes, Alzheimer's would be a factor but that realization allowed me to move forward knowing that Alzheimer's might not have the final say in Dad's story.

> There are two primary choices in life:
> to accept conditions as they exist
> or accept the responsibility
> for changing them.
> Denis Waitley

I stood up, shook myself off, and decided to fight against the darkness, the taboo, the stigma, the socially assumed death sentence, but most importantly the feeling of powerlessness. With my focus on two things,

1. my understanding of the importance of maintaining a person's dignity and

2. my understanding of what my dad did for me as a child and as an adult and my willingness to do whatever was needed in return

I was able to regain my power.

There is a saying that life is 10% what happens to you and 90% how you respond to it. Alzheimer's was not going to define him in his last years. Alzheimer's is a disease, not a man.

Somehow I knew that Alzheimer's provided me with an opportunity. If I accepted the opportunity, it would show me what I was made of and who I was. In the 11th hour, faced with more than I could ever have imagined, would I rise to meet the challenge, or, to paraphrase Michael Jordan, would I just be making excuses?

So with no excuses, I knew that I was not going to buy into the stigma and statistics, that I was in uncharted territory and that I was not going to lose my dad!

Just do
what must be done.
George Bernard Shaw

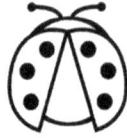

The love of family is life's greatest blessing.
Eva Burrows

Chapter 4

MOM WAS HIS ROCK ...
the foundation was set in stone

Sadly, I do not know how long my dad was treated for Alzheimer's before my mom told me the diagnosis. I know that when she did tell people, it was only her sister, my sisters and me, not even her cousin and only other blood relative, or her best friend of 70+ years. She was afraid that anyone else, anyone who loved Dad less than we did, would assume the stigma and look at him as less. She protected his privacy and his dignity.

For nearly nine years, Mom singlehandedly oversaw Dad's independence, safety, socialization, medications and environment. She worked hard to keep things "normal" and to keep Dad doing as much as reasonably possible for as long as possible. My mom was extremely successful in managing my dad's Alzheimer's by keeping his environment consistent and calm. She was his primary caregiver for the first nine years, after which she oversaw the care and my sisters and I managed it.

Mom set the tone, the attitude and the philosophy, and once my sisters and I were aware of the diagnosis, we simply followed right along in Mom's footsteps. From her nine years of navigating Alzheimer's, she taught us how to anticipate events logistically and environmentally and to pre-empt situations that might be stressful or detrimental to the needs of someone with Alzheimer's.

Once Mom experienced her medical crisis, and my sisters and I willingly accepted responsibility for managing Dad's care, we quickly learned that without our awareness she had put into action a philosophy, a goal and a strategy for dealing with early Alzheimer's that would be expanded as the disease progressed. I cannot imagine the grief and fear generated by the thought that the man Mom had loved for all but 20 years of her life was going to be "diminished" by Alzheimer's right in front of her eyes. Amid her new reality, Mom brilliantly navigated the diagnosis and the first years of symptoms and treatments. Put simply, Mom set the foundation in stone for everything that would follow.

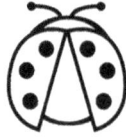

The best we can do is to help the person
to continue to live a life with
dignity, meaning and
love.
Trish Laub

Chapter 5

MY EXPERIENCE WITH EARLY ALZHEIMER'S ...
it's a disease not an identity

Shortly before I moved to Denver and began providing care for my dad, a friend asked for any insight I could offer as to my experience with my dad and Alzheimer's. My family had been dealing with Alzheimer's for about ten years when I wrote the following.

Written November 20, 2011

There is no guidebook that I know of, and every situation is different, but I have learned, and live by, the following:

1. **Let go of expecting them to be as they used to be.** They are who they are today which is *not less, just different,* than before. They **are** still in there. You can see it in their eyes, even when they appear not to remember. They are thinking and need to engage and interact.

2. **Meet them wherever they are on each day.** They may be remembering the past or repeating the same thing over and over today, or they may be in a different place. Some days they remember, some they don't. They remember a lot, and you can have conversations about whatever they remember at the time. They are on a wild ride, so go with them wherever they lead even if it makes no sense to you. It's a lot like improvisation.

3. **Don't take it personally.** Alzheimer's is "easy" on them, hard on us. They are generally happy, remember that!

They may not remember your name, but they remember you. It is hard to experience that, but it is not important whether or not they know your name or even say that they remember you. It is the connection with you that they will remember and that they need. Alzheimer's makes some people mean/angry/nasty. Again, it's not personal. It is a disease that destroys the brain! Sometimes it might be more productive to have someone else, who is not emotionally invested, interact with the person. No guilt, it might be what is best for everyone.

That said, let me just say that … Alzheimer's sucks! It is a horrible disease. My attitude is that the best that we can do is to help the person to continue to live a life with dignity, meaning and love.

Some people I know say that they either can't or don't have anything to talk about with the person. If they let go of expecting the person to be as they were before and meet the person wherever they are on that day, there will be no problem talking with the person!

Alzheimer's requires an amazing amount of patience. With children, we find boundless patience, because we understand that they don't always know what they need to do or how to do it. Not so with an adult. We expect them to know because they did at one point in time. Patience comes from your love for them and the understanding that in a way they are reversing the process of learning. They will ask the same question 1,000 times in a row, just like a child, and you need to answer the 1,000th time as patiently as you did the first. Think of a two-year-old who continually asks "Why?" If someone with Alzheimer's fixates on something, whether our reality or not, redirect them as you would a child. Ultimately, they will become in many ways like a toddler, requiring constant attention, explanation, direction and supervision. The trick is to provide it while allowing them to maintain their dignity and to feel in control. Being pre-emptive, anticipating and avoiding the next obstacle, is helpful in preventing injury, embarrassment and loss of dignity.

For me, the hardest part was when my dad knew there was something happening to him and didn't remember how things had been; he would become frustrated, embarrassed and scared. Once the person no longer recognizes that something is wrong, they are "fine." They don't even realize that they have a problem. Then it is hard only on their family. Sometimes I think at this stage, they are happier than us; they have let go of most of the things that aren't important in life.

For me, the difference between other forms of dementia and Alzheimer's is the person's ability to sequence a process. Alzheimer's destroys the brain's ability to process a sequence of tasks – which starts with not knowing in what order to do things to achieve an outcome and eventually results in not being able to eat or dress. For example, if they knock over a glass of liquid, they may look at it and not know to either get something to wipe it up or even to call someone for help. It is not that they don't care about it, but rather that they truly do not know what to do.

The last untold "jewel" of Alzheimer's is a set of symptoms called sundowning. It starts at sundown and lasts until morning. You can see it physically set in as the sun goes down. The person becomes agitated, and their movement becomes rigid. It's as though they can't sit still, can't stay in their own skin. If they sit, they want to walk. If they walk, they want to sit. They can't stay in bed, but instead wander and seem almost panicked. (More about sundowning in Chapter 6.)

My dad has been on Aricept (Donepezil) for Alzheimer's for nearly a decade. We can only assume that it helps because, going on 11 years with obvious symptoms, the disease has progressed but not nearly as quickly as in others I have known. He also takes Ativan to keep the sundowning at bay. It is sometimes effective, sometimes not as much. If he has a virus or flu bug, all of the symptoms are magnified.

My family chose to fight to keep the memories alive with a digital slideshow picture frame full of family photos and family videos. Skype and FaceTime are helpful visual alternatives to a phone call.

There are many devices available to assist with their safety as they progress. The Alzheimer's store, www.alzstore.com, is helpful.

The above, written for a friend, was my experience, understanding and perspective during early Alzheimer's. With more experience, a few of my perspectives changed.

Little did I know what lay ahead when the natural aging process was layered on top of an already challenging disease.

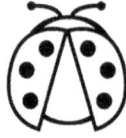

A patient advocate
is a person who
acts as the quarterback
of a care team,
coordinating the care and
protecting the rights of
a person in need of care.
Trish Laub

If you learn only one thing from this book series,
learn the need for
constant patient advocacy!

Chapter 6

OUR STORY ...
Alzheimer's and patient advocacy

While the details of this topic are elaborated upon in *Through the Rabbit Hole,* a summary of the story with my dad is presented here. All patients need an advocate, but none more than those with Alzheimer's; those often unable to advocate for themselves; those for whom even a slight change can be exponentially disruptive; and who are most often misunderstood, even disregarded.

Our Introduction to Sundowning and the Need for Patient Advocacy
I went to visit my parents in the early fall of 2007. Dad didn't seem to be feeling well but said that nothing in particular was wrong. He had lost his appetite, so Mom and I took him to dinner to entice him with a burger and, as a special treat due to his medication regime, a beer. He wasn't hungry and didn't want the beer! That's when we took him to urgent care. Fast forward, and he was taken by ambulance to the hospital due to his dangerously low heart rate.

I offered to stay overnight with Dad so that Mom could go home and sleep, as the following day would likely need her rested. Mom had been gone only a few minutes before the nurse asked a question regarding Dad's medical information for which I had no answers. It was my first encounter with needing to know medical/emergency information about Dad. Not feeling well and in an unfamiliar environment, Dad was awake nearly all night with me by his side to see that he did not get hurt while he constantly got in and out of bed. He was agitated and simply couldn't seem to sit still. Being awake all night, Dad was tired and wanted to sleep all day.

The next morning Dad had a pacemaker put in his chest. He came out of surgery and looked *pink*. I had not noticed that Dad had been literally gray due to lack of oxygen. We had to stay in the hospital another day or so and then took Dad home. The additional nights and the first night at home were challenging. He was up and down, in and out of bed, all night long.

The first night at home I slept on my parents' bedroom floor, to be available for Dad while allowing Mom to sleep. My sister covered the next night with the same experience of Dad not being able to settle down. By the third night, I called my sister in for backup. We spent the entire night awake with Dad. He would sit down, then say he had to stand up, then wanted to lay down, but seconds later he needed to walk, and on it went. It was as though he couldn't stand to be in his own skin. During that night, my sister and I agreed that we needed to go back to the hospital and find out what was happening to Dad.

We sat in the emergency room for hours while the doctors evaluated him. In the end, the diagnosis was a "jewel" of a symptom of Alzheimer's. No one in my family had ever heard of sundowning. We were blindsided by a surprise and were being introduced to it intimately. We were sent home with a medication called Ativan and told to give it to him at the first signs of sundowning.

For a couple of days, we waited to see symptoms before we gave him any medication. It wasn't a great plan as it seemed like once the symptoms got started, we couldn't get ahead of them with the medication. Inevitably, the night did not go well. We were cautious about overmedicating Dad, as it seemed that just a little too much would cause him to stay in bed all day.

One afternoon I was standing in my parents' kitchen and looked over at Dad reading the newspaper at the kitchen table. Literally, as the clock changed to 5 p.m., at sundown, something happened. I could see it happen to Dad. His face hardened, his body shifted, and it was as if something took over his nervous system. It was then that I knew that we would have to schedule his anti-sundowner's medication so that we could stay ahead of the symptoms. The Ativan schedule worked well for many years. After that, we would occasionally have to administer the medication during the day when sundowning would kick off early. This most often occurred when Dad had a secondary illness such as a cold, which seemed to disrupt his whole pattern.

When I look back, I realize that this was my family's introduction to **patient advocacy**. My dad, even though still intelligible and articulate, simply could not express what was happening inside his body. We knew something was wrong, and we had to take the steps necessary to communicate what Dad and all of us were experiencing in order to get him help and relief. We, my family and I, had to be Dad's voice. We were eventually able to get Dad to verbalize that he felt "jittery" when he was beginning to sundown. This was immensely helpful in identifying when Dad said he "didn't feel good" whether it was sundowning or something else.

The Crisis

The moving truck had left my new home in Denver, and I had embarked on a trip to Spain. Within 48 hours of my departure, Dad had unexpected surgery, which for a person with Alzheimer's is never as simple as "minor" surgery. The surgery went as expected; Dad left the hospital under his own volition and the odyssey began. Five days after arriving at skilled rehab, Dad was wearing an adult diaper and unable to communicate clearly or function properly. Relocating Dad to a second facility, it took nearly eight weeks to "detox" the damage from the first facility while my family proactively advocated for Dad at the second facility. A projected five-day skilled rehabilitation process turned into 63 days of sheer uncharted hell. The following is a *very brief summary* of the highlights of those days during which Dad was with a family member or family-sanctioned caregiver 24x7.

- Dad was **administered a pain medication that no one in our bloodline should ever be given**. No question was asked about that prior to prescribing it to him.
- The **medication made him "psychotic,"** so he was given a **sedative**.
- The **staff was uninformed** as to his specific needs and lifted him not only by the leg that had surgery but also by the arm in which he had a PICC line, a percutaneous intravenous tube, inserted. The pain caused by being moved inappropriately made him angry. More sedative.
- Dad had an **adverse reaction to the sedative,** so antipsychotic medication was prescribed.
- The medications kept him awake all night, so he **got *no* rest**.

- He required assistance going to the bathroom and *had to wait 40-60 minutes* each time before someone arrived to help. To address the delay, Dad was **made to wear adult diapers, causing heat rash and a urinary tract infection (UTI).**
- Doctor evaluation and medical **oversight were virtually nonexistent.** Also, no family meeting was held.
- **We had to come up with solutions to problems** such as having Dad wear a long-sleeved shirt from home to prevent him from pulling his PICC line out again. We also created signs notifying the staff of Dad's specific issues.
- Mom and Dad's **rights were violated** in regard to treatment which was administered with no patient/power of attorney approval.
- Dad was **severely mis-medicated and overmedicated**.
- Dad was **used in an attempt to commit Medicare fraud** by stating that he had diagnoses that he did not.
- **Safety protocols were not followed** in the facilities, putting the patients at risk.
- **Dad's safety oversight was inadequate,** even in an Alzheimer's certified facility.
- **Dad had reactions to medications** that not only caused very unpleasant behavioral changes but also almost cost him his life. My family identified those reactions and saved his life.
- **Dad was literally kidnapped**, literally. Against Mom's direction and her will, Dad was removed from the facility for an appointment.
- **We had to rent our own durable equipment** when it was needed to improve his recovery
- **Discharge was disorganized**: no doctor involvement, another patient's medications were given to us, and no prescriptions for the correct medications were written.

In summary, Dad was **almost killed due to medical error: 4 times in 63 days.**

All of this is summarized, *yes summarized*, to make a point. Sadly, this is all true. You simply cannot make this stuff up, and I have dozens of examples. Keep in mind that all of this happened in a single, nine-week, crisis. And, in a facility that was top rated, not only for Alzheimer's care but also for skilled rehab, and which was significantly better than the first facility. Overall, as was our continued experience, for the most part the RNs and CNAs were very good, but the administration involvement was counterproductive and doctor oversight was all but nonexistent. And know that we did address every grueling issue with the then new director of the facility, not only when he assumed command, but also when and after Dad was discharged.

I would like to be able to say that our experience was one in a million or even unusual, but that is not true. It is more the norm than not. We were advised and chose not to file a complaint with the state. As a family, we chose to put all of our energy into getting Dad back to himself. This is the *tip of the iceberg*. We had issues similar to those identified above at every facility, whether hospital, ER, skilled nursing or skilled rehab. However, this chapter is not specifically about being in a facility, nor the full chapter on the need for patient advocacy and approaches, both of which are covered in *Through the Rabbit Hole*. *This chapter is included to emphasize the need for patient advocacy, particularly when dealing with Alzheimer's.*

🐞🐞🐞 **Constant** oversight and patient advocacy are necessary for anyone with Alzheimer's in a medical facility, especially if they cannot advocate for themselves. Every item listed above sent Dad into "tilt" and further down into a place he did not know, and it was terrifying for him!

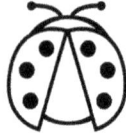

Success is simply
the achievement of a set goal.
To achieve a goal,
identify your *philosophy*,
define your *goal*
and
detail your *strategy*.
Trish Laub

Chapter 7

MY FAMILY'S PHILOSOPHY ...
Dad's still here

With any challenging situation, it is important to look at it closely and identify what you believe to be true. Without a philosophy, there can be no direction, no strategy and therefore no achievement of a goal. My family's set of beliefs became our philosophy: the basis of the strategy we used to achieve our ultimate goal.

What follows is the recollection of a nurse about a conversation with a man whose wife was living with Alzheimer's. It expresses what my family believed to be true about our dad.

He May Not Know Us, But We Still Know Who He Is
It was a busy morning, about 8:30, when an elderly gentleman in his 80s arrived at the hospital to have stitches removed from his thumb. He said he was in a hurry as he had an appointment at 9 a.m.

The nurse took his vital signs and told him to take a seat, knowing it would be over an hour before someone would be able to see him. I saw him looking at his watch and decided since I was not busy with another patient, I would evaluate his wound.

On exam, it was well healed, so I talked to one of the doctors, got the needed supplies to remove his sutures and redress his wound. While taking care of his wound, I asked him if he had another doctor's appointment this morning, as he was in such a hurry. The gentleman told me no, that he needed to go to the nursing home to eat breakfast with his wife.

I inquired as to her health. He told me that she had been there for a while and that she was a victim of Alzheimer's disease. As we talked, I asked if she would be upset if he were a bit late.

He replied that she no longer knew who he was; she had not recognized him in five years now. I was surprised, and asked him, 'And you still go every morning, even though she doesn't know who you are?'

He smiled as he patted my hand and said, 'She doesn't know me, but I still know who she is.'
Author: Unknown

No one had to say it. We all knew that eventually Dad may not remember who we were or even who he was, but we remembered, and that's all that mattered. Our dad was and always would be our dad, and we needed no other reason to continue to love and protect him. He was also a husband, a father, a grandfather, a great-grandfather and a friend to many. He was intelligent, successful, skilled, creative, and more importantly, kind, patient, loving and an extremely good man.

He was not Alzheimer's.

We were his Guardians

We were his guardians, and that role was multifaceted. The responsibility included being his voice, his advocates and his anchors to a world that became increasingly puzzling to him.

Shortly after assuming more care responsibilities for my dad, I made my dad a promise: I would keep him safe at all costs; no one would ever harm, mistreat or disrespect him. With the help of my family, I delivered on that promise.

The Golden Rule

My family lived by the Golden Rule:

> Do unto others
> as you would have them do unto you.
> adage

A good rule of thumb is to ask yourself, "*Would I like this?*" That applies to everything from meals to caregivers' treatment to the cleanliness of pajamas and bedding.

It was important to know what was important to *him*! My dad prided himself in always presenting himself as well-groomed and properly dressed. He always opted for button-down shirts and trousers rather than a t-shirt and jeans.

We did things his way, even if it required more work on our part or did not really make sense to us. It was important to Dad. It was part of respecting who he was and helped to preserve his dignity and his identity.

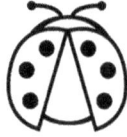

Not dying is not the same as living.
There must be meaning
for there to be life.
Trish Laub

Chapter 8

THE ULTIMATE GOAL ...
quality not quantity

Once we had a set of beliefs that defined our philosophy, my family identified our goal. While my family didn't ever want to lose Dad, the only objective was to maintain quality of life, not longevity without quality.

One day my dad might not remember the life that he had in the past, but we would protect the life of quality, meaning and love in his present. We would make the best of a potentially "bad situation" and protect the quality of every aspect of his life.

This goal of quality affected every decision that was made, especially regarding medical treatment. We knew that if we could no longer guarantee Dad's quality of life, we would assure him that it was ok for him to leave us.

It was important for us to define what quality of life meant for Dad. The three top-tier elements were safety, wellness and comfort in his care.

Also of paramount importance for his quality of life was to maintain, to the greatest extent possible, his dignity, independence, self-respect and self-worth.

Finally, we would empower him by offering him respect, a sense of purpose and love.

These requirements applied to everyone: family, our caregivers and all (physicians and those in hospitals and facilities) who worked with my dad.

47

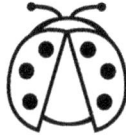

People living with Alzheimer's still have
90 billion, 80 billion, or 70 billion
active brain cells.
Those cells hold memories,
the ability to learn,
the ability to be creative
and to enjoy life.
Alzheimer's disease damages the brain,
but a lot of the brain still functions.
Those cells hold hope.

John Zeisel from *I'm Still Here*

Chapter 9

UNDERSTANDING ALZHEIMER'S ...
possibly the most important chapter

👀 👀 👀 I'm just going to say it: this may be the most important chapter of the book!

In the old days, no one knew what Alzheimer's was. Granny came to live with the family and was a little "senile." The family kept her at home so that she would be safe and no one thought much of it. Today there is a stigma associated with the disease. The stigma, that Alzheimer's is a death sentence and that the person is somehow less, is based on a lack of knowledge and resultant fear ... and it needs to change. My own mom didn't want anyone to know that Dad was living with Alzheimer's, because she feared that others would see him as less. That's not ok.

There is a lot of **fear** surrounding the dreaded disease. Some people fear being diagnosed with it, others fear a loved one having it and what they think that means. Fear is caused by not knowing the facts and falling prey to the myths.

Understanding Alzheimer's is important. Why? Because knowledge is power; knowledge empowers you with a clear understanding of what you are facing and reduces fear so you can analyze your options with a clear head and make educated decisions.

Facing the Facts

Fact #1: <u>Alzheimer's can't truly be diagnosed.</u>

The only definitive way to diagnose the disease is through an autopsy. Therefore, Alzheimer's is "diagnosed" by:

1. Medical tests such as MRIs and CT scans

2. Testing cognitive ability (which, as the disease progresses, I highly discourage!)

3. Observing physical and mental symptoms
    Physical symptoms include changes in balance, tremors (Parkinson's-like), overeating (in small part due to forgetting they ate but mostly because of damage to the area of the brain that triggers satiety) and later sundowning (come sundown, they are crawling out of their own skin).

    Mental symptoms vary but often include: confusion; loss of their sense of time and space – literally getting lost; agitation; repetition of thoughts, questions, and stories; loss of ability to remember how to process sequences (eg. using the remote); vacant looks; withdrawal; and depression.

    With many forms of dementia, the situation may elicit the words, "I forgot." With Alzheimer's, it's "I don't know" and "What's next?" Caused by a sticky plaque in the brain, in addition to a memory not existing, there is a loss of the ability to sequence simple tasks into a process.

Fact #2: <u>No one knows what causes it</u>, pure and simple.
There are theories: genetics- which is always a terrifying and
touchy subject, toxins – any number of them entering our
bodies in any number of ways (preservatives, artificial
sweeteners, heavy metals), sugar and most recently Type III
Diabetes. On a slightly comforting note, in *The Spectrum of
Hope: An Optimistic and New Approach to Alzheimer's
Disease and Dementias*, Dr. Gayatri Devi states that only 5%
of Alzheimer's diagnoses are truly genetic.

Fact #3: <u>No one knows how to prevent it</u>.
Every day I work to prevent having Alzheimer's by doing
what is believed to be healthy for our bodies and our minds.
Again, Devi states that a healthy lifestyle would prevent 60%
of all Alzheimer's diagnoses. She identifies these 6 factors as
being critical.

1. Maintaining a Healthy Weight
Maintaining a healthy weight with a BMI of 24 or less. This
helps to maintain balance in the body.

2. Treating Illness
It is important to treat any illness or disease, such as high
blood pressure or diabetes, in order to bring the body back
to optimal balance.

3. Diet
The word does not mean restriction or elimination. It
literally means "way of life." I subscribe to the pioneer diet:
fresh fruits, vegetables and proteins, with flour and sugar as
though they are in limited supply, very expensive and/or a
treat. And fluids, lots of clear pure fluids. Devi believes in a
heart healthy, not extreme, diet similar to the Mediterranean
diet and allows for limited alcohol, if desired.

4. Physical Exercise

The benefits of 30 minutes of exercise, 3 times a week to keep the body's system working at peak performance have long been known. More recently, the benefits of mindful movement are being promoted. For example, working to improve my balance and strengthening my body will help to battle the physical symptoms of Alzheimer's.

5. Brain Exercises

Use it or lose it.

Devi says, "The brain is an organ that embraces the concept of 'learned non-use.' The less you use a certain part of the brain, the less likely you are to use it over time, the fewer connections in that circuit and the more difficult it becomes to access. Grandma was right when she said, 'Use it or lose it.'"

Devi believes in a sort of "physical therapy for the brain, based on brain exercises that fall into different categories such as language and comprehension, verbal and visual memory, visuospatial skills and abstract thinking."

Creation of new neuro-pathways.

New neuro-pathways are created by doing "new to me" activities. Activities such as learning puzzles or a new sport create new neuro-pathways until the skill is learned. Once the skill is learned, practicing it continues to be mentally stimulating but does not actively create new neuro-pathways.

A study published in the New England Journal of Medicine followed elderly subjects over an impressive 21-year period to determine which activities most improved their mental sharpness and thus staved off the debilitating effects of Alzheimer's disease.

The key to avoiding Alzheimer's, in the researchers' opinion, is to continually forge *new* neural pathways. The way to do this is to constantly challenge the mind and force it to make *split-second, rapid-fire decisions.* Each of these decisions has the effect of creating greater cognitive reserve and a more complex network of neuronal synapses. In short, the more pathways your brain has to the information stored in it, the more accessible that information becomes, and the less likely you are to forget it.

The activities included leisure activities such as reading and writing as well as physical activities. Doing crossword puzzles produced a 47% lower risk of Alzheimer's while reading books produced a 35% lower risk. Surprisingly, several forms of exercise such as swimming, bicycling and playing golf produced a 0% lower risk of Alzheimer's.

👀 👀 👀 The biggest surprise was that regularly participating in dancing produced a 76% lower risk of Alzheimer's. Why dance? Partnering requires cooperation, improvisation requires rapid-fire decisions and mindful movement requires acute awareness, in the form of attention to detail, to make conscious choices.

Yes, I do dance! I'm stacking my deck the best I can to avoid having Alzheimer's.

6. Social Engagement
A combination of physical and mental activity experienced through stimulating activities and social interaction help to maintain the brain's vitality. Social engagement results in improved mood, helps meet the emotional need for companionship and promotes independence.

In addition to Devi's recommendation, I believe that you should <u>do what makes you feel alive</u> so that it becomes cellular.

What is the name of your favorite song? Can you speak the lyrics? If I were to put on the song, could you sing the lyrics? That's cellular memory.

As I mentioned previously, my dad is in the University of Denver Hall of Fame for both basketball and tennis. Within a year prior to his passing, a caregiver arrived at his home with an orange rubber ball. She tossed it to Dad, and in his delight he began to handle his perceived basketball, skillfully threading it around his back and through his legs as though he was on the basketball court. It had likely been decades since he had played the game, but the cellular memory caused by years of repetition remained.

That cellular memory can be invaluable for someone with Alzheimer's, triggering the joy of the memory, and in this case, initiating physical activity.

I am also working on being <u>a better, kinder person</u>. There is a thought that Alzheimer's amplifies a person's basic being. If that is the case, I want to be kinder, not angrier.

Alanna Shaikh, in her Ted talk on Alzheimer's, said this about her dad: "When you take away everything he ever learned in this world, his naked heart still shines. I need a heart so pure that if it's stripped bare by dementia it will survive."

Fact #4: <u>What I **do** know</u> … is that a meaningful life is possible with Alzheimer's.

Dispelling Some Myths

Alzheimer's is another stage in life, no less valuable than all the other stages. We don't know what my dad's or my family's lives would have been like, healthy or not, had Alzheimer's not been a part of it. While no one wants to hear the diagnosis of Alzheimer's, understanding what Alzheimer's is and is not will help you to find perspective. Whether people view the situation positively or negatively has a major impact on the success of the person receiving the diagnosis to live with the illness.

The myths are caused by ignorance, in the literal definition of the word meaning "a lack of knowledge," about Alzheimer's. There are several Alzheimer's myths that propagate fear. Where do the myths come from? They are derived from outdated information, before the importance of diet, supplementation, exercise and brain stimulation were understood. Additionally, we live in a culture where few truly understand Alzheimer's and even fewer want to talk about it.

Myth #1: <u>Alzheimer's is always a death sentence which ends in a nursing home.</u>
False. Alzheimer's is viewed as a life-limiting disease. It is an accelerated aging of the brain. If no other pre-existing condition, such as heart disease or diabetes, ultimately causes death, the symptoms of Alzheimer's may result in death at some point. According to the Mayo Clinic, those diagnosed with Alzheimer's usually live from 8-10 to as long as 20 years, most of which are often lived independently. The truth is, that for many, the symptoms of Alzheimer's are not the cause of death. For others, the aging of the brain caused

by Alzheimer's will be the cause of death in the same way that the natural aging of the brain and other organs cause death.

The death-sentence myth has expanded into the **false** thought that all affected by Alzheimer's end up in nursing homes unable to know their surroundings and circumstances, and unable to function. Alzheimer's has been defined as a "spectrum disease," meaning that every case of Alzheimer's is different and that success in treatment is based on person-centered care. A small percentage of Alzheimer's cases end in a nursing home out of necessity.

Myth #2: <u>Alzheimer's is not treatable or curable</u>.
It is *true* that at this point, Alzheimer's is not curable. It is, however, *false* that is it not treatable, meaning that the impairment and symptoms can be alleviated.

Alzheimer's treatment has been found effective in stopping the progression. Because Alzheimer's is treatable, it is critical to have a "treatment approach," one that includes pharmacological and nonpharmacological options.

Myth #3: <u>A person living with Alzheimer's has lost all memory.</u>
False. It is helpful to have a conceptual understanding of how our memories are stored. In *Contented Dementia*, author Oliver James writes about the person-centered approach to Alzheimer's care developed by Penelope Garner, called SPECAL (Specialized Early Care for Alzheimer's). To help others better understand Alzheimer's, Garner uses the analogy of a photo album to describe the manner in which we store our memories. She says that normally each page stores a memory, and on that page are factual data, including images, about the memory and a record of the emotions

attached to the memory. The memories that were created prior to the onset of Alzheimer's are intact, like a page of the photo album just described. These memories are very helpful in anchoring the person to our reality. Additionally, if positive emotions are attached to the memory, it helps create a sense of well-being.

As Alzheimer's progresses, memories are stored with less of the factual data, but always all of the emotional response. This results in a photo album page being literally blank as far as some or most of the factual data. But if the page is accessed, the emotions are still there. The person does not have the actual memory but remembers the emotional response to it. So if someone is unkind to a person with Alzheimer's, they may not remember the details of the incident, but they remember the way it made them feel. Sometimes they remember a bad feeling without being able to remember why.

My dad was able to create some sort of new memories. We had 17 caregivers in 18 months, ending with a dream team of seven caregivers. He "knew" all of his caregivers, as being part of his safe "tribe," although he did not know the names of all of them. He did begin to associate the name with the caregiver when we used it. Two of his caregivers were young identical twin males, who were difficult for even my family members to differentiate. Dad could tell the two apart and associate their names with them. I don't know if that was because he attached the warm, loving feelings he received from them to each twin. But he definitely learned and knew who they each were.

It is true that Dad could not learn new sequences, but he seemed to be able to create a type of memory of each caregiver based on how they made him feel.

Myth #4: <u>We are lost to those with Alzheimer's and they to us</u>.

This simply is *false*. Alzheimer's diminishes the memory; it does not take away the relationships, the experiences or the emotions of those memories. And, more of the brain works than does not. In fact, the brain still contains billions of working cells. In spite of the disease, most individuals are exceptionally perceptive, creative and highly emotionally aware. They are not lost, only unfamiliar with their new circumstances. They are the same individual as before the diagnosis and possibly more in need of our connection. As long as we focus on their assets, as opposed to their deficits, they will continue to remain connected to us. We are their anchor. The truth is that with continued deterioration there is an increase in their need for human connection, compassion, patience and love, as they have heightened susceptibility to isolation and sensitivity to disrespect.

Myth #5: <u>As the illness progresses, the individual ceases to be a person</u>.

False. Does a person have to be articulate, intelligible, remember our name or function independently in order to be a person? Of course not. As a culture, we assist and support those living with disabilities who may have far greater limitations than those caused by Alzheimer's, but we do not do the same for those with Alzheimer's.

Everyone has their unique capabilities. It is our job to identify and focus on them so that everyone living with Alzheimer's, no matter where in the progression of the disease they are, maintains their dignity and self-respect.

Myth #6 Underline: People with Alzheimer's become mean and aggressive.
Absolutely false. This is the most frustrating myth for me. It requires a *thorough* understanding of the following section.

🐞 🐞 🐞 Neither aggression nor nastiness is a symptom of Alzheimer's. That does not mean that an individual with Alzheimer's will not exhibit those behaviors. If they do, it is not a symptom of the disease. See the following section for clarification of this myth.

🐞

The True Symptoms of Alzheimer's

The most helpful description of Alzheimer's symptoms is found in the book *I'm Still Here, A New Philosophy of Alzheimer's Care* by John Zeisel. Here is my interpretation adapted from Mr. Zeisel's description.

When someone has a knee injury (disease) and loses the function of their leg (primary symptom), they may overuse it and cause it to hurt (secondary side effect) resulting in irritability (secondary behavior). Additional pain and irritability are not symptoms of the knee injury, and we do not say that they are.

When someone with Alzheimer's is nasty or irritable, we blame Alzheimer's and the person for their behavior rather than looking at the causes. Understanding primary symptoms and secondary side effects and behaviors is critical in identifying what is happening. With that knowledge, everyone involved can make the best-possible treatment decisions.

Regarding Alzheimer's:

Primary symptoms are directly attributed to either cognitive or executive functional impairment, such as the inability to access memories or organize complex thoughts or tasks, caused by the damage in the brain from Alzheimer's.

Secondary side effects or behaviors, such as frustration and yelling, are consequences of untreated primary symptoms. It is not a symptom of the illness; it is a *reaction* to a symptom of the illness. It may be a result of an inability to process external stimuli such as a violent TV show, too much noise, an unfamiliar environment, or too many verbal commands. Removal of the stimuli may cease the behavior (yelling) or side effect (frustration) or may not.

👀👀👀 **Unrelated behaviors** are behaviors that are not reactions to the symptoms of Alzheimer's. They are often mistaken as symptoms but are reasonable reactions that would have occurred had the person not had Alzheimer's. They are most often caused by negative personal interaction such as being rushed or disrespected or an adverse reaction to medications.

👀👀👀 Aggression is almost never a primary symptom of Alzheimer's. It may be a secondary or an unrelated behavior caused by unmet needs that may include an inability to express those needs, inappropriate environment, perceived aggression, or negative personal interactions. These are all situations in which the person might have reacted aggressively had they not had Alzheimer's. Now, please read that again!

For example, the *physical manifestation of the primary condition* is damage to the brain that causes cognitive or functional impairments: being able to access memories or organize complex thoughts or tasks.

The *primary symptoms* of the disease are a direct result of the damage to the brain, for example, inability to process complex tasks and loss of impulse control.

Feeling confused in complex situations and reacting to that feeling in a negative manner, resulting in irritation and aggression, are *secondary side effects and behaviors.* These may further result in withdrawal and apathy.

If during the course of a day, someone speaks disrespectfully or a caregiver accidently causes pain to the person, they may react with aggression that is a *behavior unrelated* to Alzheimer's.

How understanding the symptoms is helpful:
The person with Alzheimer's has the flu and therefore needs assistance transferring from chair to bed. They are confused as to the need for assistance and do not process the need. They may first resist the need, which may escalate to combativeness, as they feel the visceral reaction to defend themself against the perceived violation against them. It may trigger anger, fear and anxiety, and while these are not symptoms of Alzheimer's, they aren't helpful to the situation.

This situation can be avoided by recognizing the stimuli (the perception that assistance is not needed) for the initial resistance and stopping the process. Walk away, if possible, and re-enter as though starting over. Most of the time the individual will not remember the situation unless it emotionally escalated. Return and ask if assistance is wanted. If the response is positive, ask permission to assist. If the response is negative, offer assistance. If it is declined, do your best to keep the individual safe while they try to execute the move. When they see that they need assistance, you can calmly begin the process again.

👀 👀 👀 In each of the few instances in which Dad either said something seemingly unkind or expressed himself physically, I can honestly say that the behavior was caused by negative personal interactions. Once the stimulus was identified and was removed, the negative behavior disappeared. That said, if someone mistreated him, he did not forget, and in fact remembered every time they entered the room. There are many potential external stimuli such as inappropriate treatment by anyone, especially caregivers, inadequate time allowed for tasks or insufficient planning for events, to name a few.

Conditions secondary to Alzheimer's, such previously existing conditions or an illness can make the primary condition more severe than it is by itself. With Alzheimer's this seems to be particularly true. My dad had a hip that should have been replaced years before he needed caregiving. The hip impeded his ability to walk, and therefore made the process of navigating movement more of a complex skill causing more frustration and agitation. There are also illnesses that, as a temporary secondary condition, worsen the symptoms and behaviors of Alzheimer's such as pneumonia, UTIs (Urinary Tract Infections), fevers, colds and sinus infections. In addition, adverse reactions to medicine and unaddressed issues of visual impairment or hearing loss can generate problems including: discomfort, dizziness, pain, heightened agitation and loss of balance. It is as though the individual has gone into "tilt" and everything is amplified. Finally, the natural aging process is also such a condition.

A Necessary and Effective Treatment Approach
According to the Oxford Dictionary, treatment means *the manner in which someone behaves toward or deals with someone or something.* First and foremost, everyone should be treated as a person.

In the treatment of the person, it is important to fully understand the previous section, **The True Symptoms of Alzheimer's,** which explains primary symptoms, secondary side effects and behaviors and unrelated behaviors. Once those are understood, it becomes possible to develop a strategy for avoiding negative or unwanted behaviors, which impede treatment of the primary symptoms.

Evaluate – Modify – Treat

1. Evaluate the current situation.
What is the behavior and what are the possible immediate causes? Are there external stimuli that may trigger a negative response? Is the room too cold or is there too much noise or activity in the room that might cause agitation? Is there a lack of space in which to move, causing a feeling of insecurity? Has someone been impatient and caused a sense of being rushed? If no external stimuli can be identified, has there been a change in routine? Has there been a medication change? Have there been any other changes?

Also evaluate the following 4 As, as identified by John Zeisel in *I'm Still Here: A New Philosophy of Alzheimer's Care*:

- Apathy may be caused by the inability to perceive the future and therefore to plan, resulting in a lack of stimulation.
- Anxiety can come from insecurity due to the lack of a sense of time and unfamiliarity with relationships.
- Agitation is likely due to overstimulation, frustration or the inability to initiate activity.
- Aggression is an uncontrolled reaction to what is happening due to the inability to control impulses, which is caused by the disease.

2. Modify the situation.
While evaluating and identifying, discontinue anything that may be contributing to the problem behavior. If possible, leave the room, allowing time for the person to "reset," then re-enter and start again.

For example, if someone doesn't want a bath and is angry about having to take one, you might remind them that they like to be clean and encourage them to do the task. Finesse goes a long way.

3. Treat appropriately.
If modification of the situation does not resolve the problem, treat.

In this approach, we first treat the person, then the illness. To treat also means to alleviate symptoms and to promote healing. Treating the person first puts us in the best position to then treat the illness. Doing everything we can to see that the environment and routine are most conducive to the comfort of the person, allows us to evaluate what symptoms need to be treated further.

There are many Nonpharmacological treatments available which are helpful to those with Alzheimer's:

- Managing their environment and helping them be in control of it
- Subtly helping them be as independent as possible by making sure that their environment is accessible and safe
- Managing their schedule, allowing enough time for all tasks and events
- Ensuring human connection, interaction and engagement. People may think that it's not useful, but people and repeated stories are critical, as memories keep them attached to life. Human touch and facial expressions will become more critical as the individual's ability to express themself, or even understand us, diminishes.
- Providing things which cue memories, such as digital photo frames and familiar music
- Waiting for them to express themself instead of speaking for them
- Nonmedicinal treatments: supplements, massage, EVOX (emotional reframing is useful in alleviating stress, anxiety, anger and emotional trauma), behavioral treatments and acupuncture to name a few

If further treatment is needed, medication can be considered *only as a last resort.*

> Medical treatment should be the servant of genuine human caring, never its master.
> William H Thomas, M.D. from *Learning from Hannah*

Pharmacological treatment
The biggest issue with pharmaceuticals is with inappropriate prescriptions, improper dosing, unacknowledged drug

interactions and unnecessarily medicating non-primary behaviors and side effects. Too often the result is a drug cocktail in which some of the drugs actually are treating side effects of earlier drugs and creating worse side effects in the process. Over the counter (OTC) medications are regulated by the Food and Drug Administration and must be considered pharmaceuticals and evaluated as such.

For example, my dad was given a pain medication that caused borderline psychotic behavior. That behavior was then treated with an anti-anxiety medication and a sedative. When the sedative caused further negative behavior, an antipsychotic medication was prescribed. When my family identified the real problem and changed the pain medication, the behavior went away. The additional medications, each with their unique side effects, were not only ineffective but also unnecessary.

If all potential sources of the issue have been identified and eliminated, and all alternative treatments have been exhausted, medications should be considered.

As with evaluating the 4 As, each issue (symptom, side effect, behavior) needs to be evaluated individually. For example, depression has been associated with Alzheimer's and many other serious and life-limiting diseases. But depression can also be the result of feeling disengaged from others and the world. If the latter sources of depression have been properly addressed and the depression persists, then an antidepressant may be appropriate. Medication should always be the last choice, not the first. Evaluate the source, modify and adjust external stimuli, treat and lastly medicate.

That said, there are pharmaceuticals that are successful in slowing the progression of Alzheimer's, reducing anxiety and sundowning symptoms, enhancing cognitive function and treating excess disabilities.

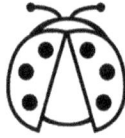

One of the happiest moments in life
is when you find the courage
to let go of what you can't change.
Unknown

Chapter 10

UNDERSTANDING A LIFE WITH ALZHEIMER'S ...
different -- not less

Once my family had a philosophy and a goal, we needed a strategy to achieve that goal. To develop the strategy, which was the nuts and bolts of his care, we had to understand what it's like to live with Alzheimer's and what is successful when working with someone with Alzheimer's.

We as a family learned a great deal about what was successful when working with my dad. We observed thousands of hours of professionals working with him and did our research, being careful that our approaches were in strict alignment with our philosophy and goal.

Because Alzheimer's causes loss of memory and ultimately independence, it can therefore result in loss of self-worth, self-respect, dignity, identity and meaning. Can you imagine how it would feel to lose even one of those elements of personhood? The battle we faced was to protect the very definition of my dad's quality of life.

The Real Killers
Another book that was enlightening is *Learning from Hannah, Secrets for a Life Worth Living* by William H Thomas, a book based on the Eden Alternative for Care. This book identifies the "three big killers" of the aging as:

helplessness, loneliness and hopelessness.

Helplessness
The greatest fears women voice about getting Alzheimer's is that they will forget their loved ones, become a burden to their families and not be able to care for themselves. While those were among Dad's biggest fears, his single greatest fear was that he could not take care of Mom. When Mom was in medical crisis, Dad would constantly ask "Is Mom ok?" and "What can I do to help her?" It was a constant task to help Dad feel self-worth by having him help all of us in any way in which he was able. The feeling of helplessness led to agitation, anxiety and loss of self-worth and self-respect.

Loneliness
At points in the life of someone with Alzheimer's, they may get lost in their own reality, their own world, which may result in isolation and withdrawal from ours. They can become overstimulated by noise and activity that they no longer understand or can tolerate. In addition, those with Alzheimer's are subject to losing the ability to socialize outside their living space, further isolating them. The need for human connection is necessary for every living being, but particularly critical for those living with Alzheimer's, as they are susceptible to losing touch with the outside world. Those with Alzheimer's are comforted by the warmth of the human connection. As their senses diminish, as in natural aging, touch, contact through the eyes, even smell become invaluable. Engaging them boosts their self-worth and promotes a sense of purpose. Without human connection, those with Alzheimer's lose their tether to reality and can become lost.

Hopelessness
Helplessness and loneliness can lead to hopelessness. Hopelessness is compounded by the difficulty with complex thoughts, which is a symptom of Alzheimer's. Dad would ask "What am I going to do?" He had the feeling that there was something he should or wanted to be doing, to feel worthy, but he did not know what it was.

The "three big killers" lead to depression, isolation, apathy, loss of self-worth and self-respect, and a lack of value in living.

A New Approach
In *I'm Still Here*, Zeisel shares the importance of:

- **Hearing and responding to the person living with Alzheimer's. First, the person's reality is real to them.** If it is scary, reassure them that they are **safe.** Do not try to convince them that their reality is not correct. Do not assume that they do not know what they are saying. Towards the end of nine weeks of skilled rehab, I asked my dad where he wanted to go. He repeatedly stated a specific location, which many suggested was NOT his actual answer. After getting the same response to that question several dozen times, it was determined that the location WAS where my dad really wanted to go.

- **Being honest.** Never lie to them, but be kind in telling them the truth.

- **Addressing them directly and looking them in the eye.** They are an individual, not to be addressed as "we." They have Alzheimer's, "we" do not.

- **Providing necessary information**. Never "test" them by asking questions such as "do you know?" Do not put them in a position to feel failure.
- **Fostering independence.** Do as little as possible for them, allow success and self-worth.
- **Diverting and redirecting.** It is important to do so without saying "don't."
- **Responding, not reacting.** If they are angry, let it go and let them regroup
- **Being present.** There is no concern other than the here and now, no rush.
- **Using all the senses.** Don't only talk: show, touch and offer taste and smell.

Along the way, we were taught that the following are also very important, which was a valuable lesson:
- Speak slowly, clearly and gently, using few words. Especially when they are "confused" or tired, <u>aim for three words</u>.
- Don't talk about them in front of them, as though they are not there.
- Be prepared to let them take as long as they want or need to do every task. They need to do as much for themselves as possible every day, or they will lose the skill.
- Keep noise to a minimum, specifically phone conversations, and the creation of multiple sounds at the same time, such as conversation and TV.
- Engage them. They know when you are there but not engaged with them.
- Always ask for their permission ("May I?") before doing <u>anything</u> to them. In order to preserve their sense of power over their life, never dictate or demand.

Let Them Take Their Time

What is specific to Alzheimer's disease, more so than any other form of dementia, is the need to let them do things in their own time. They move slowly. It can be very frustrating and requires an extra amount of patience. There is no rushing someone with Alzheimer's, as it can result in unwanted secondary side effects or behaviors.

Having Alzheimer's, it was incredibly important that Dad operated on his schedule, other than being given meds which were required at 10 a.m. and 6 p.m. Being rushed was stressful for him. He could become irritable when rushed or given too many directions, too quickly, too often. And he needed to be able to do as much as possible for himself, which took a lot of time.

Every Day is a New Day

Every couple of days were different. Some days were good, others not so much. Most nights were decent, others were tough. Sometimes Dad was in an almost "altered state," somewhere between conscious and unconscious. Whatever state he was in, that was his reality. His reality could be scary, and we would tell him that he was safe. Always, but particularly during these altered-state phases and at night, it was incredibly important to be patient with him.

Encourage Them to Do as Much as Possible

It was important to assess Dad every day to determine what he was capable of doing each day. His goal was to do as much as possible, but some days he could not do things. If he was particularly weak, it may have been best not to try to require him to do specific tasks at specific times. We had all day to complete several tasks. In a given day, the only things that were **required** to be completed were meds and hydration. It was equally important to remember that just because Dad couldn't do something one day, or for a few days, did not mean that he couldn't do it today or again in the future.

For example, Dad had exceptional small-motor skills. Therefore, we encouraged him to use that skill. Whether it was buttoning his shirts or pajamas or opening something small, we encouraged him, no matter how long it took him, to complete the task. If there was shredding to do, and Dad was capable of doing it even with assistance, the task was assigned to him. It kept him engaged with us as we collectively did projects and allowed him to be responsible for a task and feel self-worth.

Sensory Overload is a Huge Problem

Too much noise (multiple sounds, multiple conversations, too much volume, people speaking too fast, etc.) causes a person with Alzheimer's to withdraw and can make them irritable. It is important to be aware of the sounds and volume of what is going on in their environment. Placing a towel over an appliance when using it will dampen a whining sound and the volume it produces. Conducting personal phone calls in another room will eliminate that factor from the environment. Constant stimulation can be overwhelming therefore quiet time is valuable. All of this is compounded when one wears hearing aids.

The Senses

Our senses diminish as we age. Sight is usually first to diminish, followed by taste, smell and touch. Hearing is the last sense to go; even people in comas can still hear. As each sense diminishes, those that have not diminished heighten. As a person's ability to communicate falters, their sensitivity to emotions increases. They become incredibly sensitive to the positive or negative energy of other people.

> I've learned that
> people will forget what you said,
> people will forget what you did,
> but people will never forget
> how you made them feel.
> Maya Angelou

Dad "rested" a lot during the day. However, a lot of the time he was just sitting there with his eyes closed. This is a normal byproduct of Alzheimer's. Many times when his eyes were closed, he was awake and very aware of what was going on. He was able to hear phone conversations and often thought that someone was speaking to him. This was not only confusing for him, but also distressing as he was **very** sensitive to the tone of the conversation he heard. Also because he was aware of what was going on even with his eyes closed, he would feel alone if someone in the same room was not interacting with him. He loved and needed company and attention. When we rubbed his back, he felt good, and he relaxed. When someone spoke with him, he smiled and enjoyed being with them. His life was enriched by those simple acts.

As Dad's senses diminished, he couldn't always remember what someone said to him, but he always remembered the way that person made him feel.

Idiosyncrasies are Amplified

My dad didn't like being told what to do. I don't think anyone does. Things went most smoothly when he was presented with a **request**, when we **asked** what he wanted and when we asked his permission. Sometimes he needed a gentle nudging and encouragement. It was always important to protect his dignity and his right **to make the decisions that he could.**

He also did not like to be repeatedly asked questions, especially whether he was done with a meal or if he wanted to go to bed. It made him feel like he was not only being rushed and pressured, but also nagged. He needed as much time as he required to complete a task on his own.

Lessons From a Kind of _You_-topia

A lot can be learned from a special community in the Netherlands, a village specifically created to be an alternative to a nursing home and allowing those with Alzheimer's to live as independently, yet safely, as possible. It is a village where the seasons can be enjoyed, but there is only one exit, which is kept locked. The village includes a restaurant. All employees within the village are trained in Alzheimer's care.

The housing units allow for one of seven lifestyle themes attracting people with like interests, as opposed to assigning housing on a first-come first-served basis.

The objective is to create normalcy by creating a routine, and sticking to it. The stores have no prices and residents have no money, allowing them the ability to "purchase" goods without the concern of dealing with money and making change.

The village aims to provide a welcome feeling and an enjoyable life. They offer 25 clubs to keep residents active, placing a high value on music. Although they have automatic elevators, residents are invited to exercise even if only in the form of walking, with the goal of helping them to stay strong and live a healthy life. Residents are now living longer, meaningful lives, staying three years instead of two.

De Hogeweyk, aka Dementiavillage, in Weesp, Holland is an example of a special community in which the individuals are valued and assisted in living a good life.

It's not Easy

Living with or providing care for someone living with Alzheimer's is not easy. Even if you have a thorough understanding of both Alzheimer's and a life with it, and even if you have the ideal situations and do everything "right," it's still not easy. You are not a super hero with super powers, you are merely human. It is important for you, and those who support you, to be aware of the pitfalls and of when help is needed. Fatigue and hurt feelings lead to impatience, which leads only to more negative situations and from there, things spiral downward. Even when you recognize the difficulty of the situation, it doesn't mean that you can always handle it. In the end, you cannot "save," meaning make well, the person with Alzheimer's. The best you can do is to help the person to continue to live a life with dignity, meaning and love. To do so, ask yourself, "Is what I am doing helping or hurting the situation?" If you are unable to improve the situation, you need to ask for help and take a break. Take time to recharge and rejuvenate, and when you have the courage again, and it does take courage, return to dealing with Alzheimer's.

> Courage doesn't always roar.
> Sometimes courage is the quiet voice
> at the end of the day saying,
> "I will try again tomorrow."
> Mary Anne Radmacher

With aging, our verbal filters fall away, and even more so for those with Alzheimer's. Their frustration with losing context in the world, coupled with their diminishing filters, can result in negative communication such as criticism. The person with Alzheimer's may forget what they said or did that was hurtful, but remember the feeling of frustration and possibly the negative emotion they expressed. In addition, they are often incapable of "fixing" or even addressing their negative behavior. Those living with or providing care for the person are particularly susceptible to this, as they are already working hard to do their best in a challenging situation. Many are working off of their last energetic and emotional reserves and they are somewhat fragile. The recipient of the negative communication, while understanding the frustration, may still feel hurt, especially if that person is tired. The recipient remembers the incident while the other person does not. It's not easy.

As I've said, it requires an inordinate amount of patience to live with or care for someone with Alzheimer's. It is easy to be impatient. When someone with Alzheimer's requires what we deem as too much time, or are unable to complete a task, it is easy to project that impatience onto their ability to complete other tasks. None the less, it is critical that someone with Alzheimer's not only be allowed, but also encouraged, to do as much as they are capable of doing. If you find that you are losing patience, get some help and take a break. Again, it's not easy.

Family situations can be particularly challenging, especially if caregiving is necessary. There are many dynamics that come in to play and must be considered. *Through the Rabbit Hole* discusses caregiving requirements, but also the specific challenges families face.

None of it is easy, but it is worthwhile.

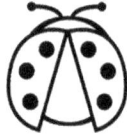

The truth is - everything counts.
Everything.
Everything we do and everything we say.
Everything helps or hurts,
everything adds to or takes away
from someone else.
Countee Cullen

Chapter 11

MY FAMILY'S STRATEGY ...

comfort in his care

According to Merriam Webster, a strategy is defined as a careful plan or method for achieving a particular goal, usually over a long period. My family's strategy was focused on person-centered care and support.

Our strategy was based on our philosophy that Dad was still capable of living a life meaningful to him and others around him. Armed with information and daily experience with Alzheimer's, we worked to ensure that every care decision upheld that philosophy.

This chapter speaks to my family's approach to caring for my dad, and is specific to our philosophy, goal and Alzheimer's. *Through the Rabbit Hole, the companion book to this one,* discusses the many aspects of care, including care options and working with caregivers. This chapter provides an additional layer of information.

My Daily Ritual

My day caring for Dad began with a ritual, one that set the tone for the day and re-established the connection between us. I would stand outside his condo door, take a deliberate breath and exhale thoughts of everything except the current moment and anything outside of his home. It was like hitting a reset button that created a calm assertiveness. This ritual allowed me to look at the new day with fresh eyes and thoughts, and to have the patience necessary to address whatever was happening inside.

Once inside, I waved hello to Mom, who knew she would receive a proper greeting later, and immediately went to wherever Dad was: bed, bathroom, kitchen bar stool, or most likely his reclining chair in the family room. Once there, I would get to his eye level, often kneeling at his recliner, and look him straight in the eyes. I would say "Hi Dad!" then point to my eyes and say "Look at my eyes, who's eyes are these?" He would look at my eyes intently, smile, and say, "Your eyes." "Yes, and they are yours, too," I would reply, because I look just like him. The connection was made.

There are various other ways to connect. I have a dear friend who found that singing the song "You are my sunshine" immediately connects her and her husband to her mother-in-law. It is not important how you do it, but rather that you make that connection.

Daily Objectives
We had very clear daily objectives. Many things might or might not have happened during a day, but our objectives were always to be met, and would be deal breakers if violated for everyone who came into contact with Dad.

Daily Objectives
Frank is safe.
Frank's meds are given correctly and on time.
Frank is clean.
Frank is fed.
Frank is happy.

These were the most basic requirements to be met by all. Ensuring Dad's safety was an obvious requirement. The proper administration of his medication was critical to maintaining balance and quality of life. When sundowning became a symptom, it was critical that his medication be given prior to the onset of the symptom, otherwise the next 18-24 hours would be very unpleasant for Dad and his caregivers. Being clean is a basic human need. Who wants to wear clothes that are dirty, possibly with food, blood, or bodily fluids, let alone to sleep on dirty sheets. Again, being fed on time and properly is a basic human requirement. And finally, ensuring that Dad was as happy as possible, given the challenges of Alzheimer's, was paramount to his quality of daily life.

Mantra

You are **safe**! As stated before, there is a great potential for fear in someone who is losing their bearings on our reality and sometimes lives in their own. "You are safe" is the sentence that will allay that fear regardless of the reality in which they are present. While "You are safe' was our mantra, the addition of "We love you" went a long way to comfort Dad.

Routine with Flexibility

When I was first told about the importance of a routine for those with Alzheimer's I kind of smiled to myself. It was in the early going, and I had already experienced that every day with Alzheimer's is different. Some days went as envisioned, and others diverged radically. I soon found a compromise between going with flow and adhering to a schedule: I adopted the consciousness of consistency with flexibility.

83

What this meant was that my family would start the day with an intended schedule, understanding that medications had to be given at specific times, and allow some flexibility in the schedule to adapt to Dad's specific needs.

We gathered knowledge on what might be important in that schedule. But understanding that things change day to day, moment to moment, we knew that we would have to let go of the "should."

It is not the strongest of the species that survives, nor the most intelligent that survives.
It is the one that is most adaptable to change.
Charles Darwin

In addition, over time things will change, maybe every couple of months or more often. There will be pajama days, those days when Dad simply couldn't seem to get out of bed or didn't want to get dressed. It usually meant that something was amiss and required some observation. On those days it was likely that he wouldn't want to eat as much and possibly needed additional oversight with his intake of liquids. Occasionally Dad's behavior or mentation (mental activity) would change, again causing a disruption in the schedule. When this happened, we would evaluate several factors: timing and dosage of his medications (always checked first), environment, care, and signs of an unrelated illness. Having any illness, no matter how minor, could set Dad into a kind of "tilt", exacerbating the symptoms of Alzheimer's, and creating a bigger challenge.

In establishing a routine, it was helpful to know exactly what Dad wanted and how he wanted it. Our work went more smoothly when we provided what Dad wanted. The days were rewarding, but could be long and grueling. Whenever it could have been easier for **me** to do something, such as let him go to bed early, I had to ask myself if it was what was best for Dad.

The bottom line is that we had a goal and created a routine that was flexible and allowed for evolution.

Patient Advocacy
As talked about previously in this book and in my other books, we are the guardians of those with Alzheimer's, their voice. The need for patient advocacy, especially for those who cannot protect themselves, is **constant**.

Know the rights of the person with Alzheimer's, as well as those of their Power of Attorney. Nothing should be done to, or changes made for, the person being treated without their consent or that of their power of attorney.

Immediately create an Emergency book, with contents including family history and up-to-date medical history. Put a spiral notebook with it for taking notes at appointments. Use a separate notebook for each medical event or facility stay. Take these books to every doctor's appointment, all Emergency Department visits and to any stays in a facility.

Create daily log sheets, highlighting the daily routine including the details of medicine administration and an area in which notes can be written. (See *Through the Rabbit Hole* for more detail.) This was immensely helpful to us in tracking any errors or changes in Dad's care.

Educate yourself, ask questions, question answers and exercise every option. We were told that Dad would have to have pureed food and thickened drinks for the rest of his life due to dysphagia. In his case, dysphagia did not present as an inability to swallow, but rather that when he did, the mechanism didn't work correctly causing him to have to clear his throat often and possibly aspirate into his lungs. This is not uncommon for those who have had anesthesia, but most often it resolves itself. With Dad it seemed to be an ongoing problem. Therefore, we followed the dysphagia protocol. (*Through the Rabbit Hole* details information on dealing with dysphagia.) At one point, three to four months prior to his passing, I noticed that he was no longer clearing his throat and it occurred to me that possibly his dysphagia had resolved to some degree. When I suggested the idea, I was told that it wasn't likely. When I requested that the benign, noninvasive and nonthreatening test be redone, the results showed that Dad's dysphagia had in fact decreased. The recommendation for food preparation was reduced to allowing sticky food, unpureed. Dad's last Thanksgiving, Christmas and New Year's Eve dinners were the same as the rest of the family. This is an example of something that Dad could not have thought of or verbalized, and that the doctors didn't think of or expect, but it increased his quality of life. It brought Dad not only great joy to eat the meals he so enjoyed but also a greater sense of normalcy. The point is: always think, ask, pursue. It is worth it. Run that extra test even if there is only .01% of 1% chance that it will improve their quality of life. The worst that anyone can say to a request is "no."

In our patient advocacy, we wanted others to recognize that Dad was a valued human being. When he was in facilities we brought a huge (2 ft. by 3 ft.) poster of family photos so that those in the facilities knew that Dad had a small army of people to whom he was important, by whom he was loved. It not only humanized Dad to the staff, but also showed him in his wholeness, as opposed to seeing him only as a patient.

Interaction

Caring for someone with Alzheimer's requires compassion. We are the guardians of their identity, their voice and their reality. It requires an understanding of Alzheimer's and of the person.

It is also critical to treat them with respect, protect their dignity, empower them, and be truthful and kind.

Empowerment allows the person to thrive even though the normal aging process is combined with Alzheimer's. We worked to allow Dad to make every decision he was capable of making for himself. Until he was unconscious in his final days, no one ever did anything for or to Dad without his prior verbal approval. It was a simple act of respect to ask Dad if he wanted help with something or if he preferred to do it himself. Dad only refused approval when he was not feeling well, and in those instances, we were able to finesse the situation to gain his permission.

Another part of empowerment was independence. Independence was part of allowing Dad to make his own decisions. It also meant that we encouraged Dad to do as much for himself as possible. Many times it would have been faster to button his shirt for him, but he continued to have exceptional small-motor skills so we patiently waited for him to button the shirt himself.

Dad was never to be lied to, **ever**! When a challenging situation arose, it was important to tell the truth in a manner that would be least stressful to him. Sometimes Dad would ask where his parents were, even though they had passed away many decades ago. I would reply that if they were still alive, they would be approximately 120 years old and that they were no longer with us. He would think about it and, while a little sad, appeared to accept it. My answer was much kinder than blurting out that they were dead, possibly causing him to grieve again and again. Another example was when Mom was hospitalized for six weeks. She was his anchor. My family was worried about the effect her absence would have on him. We worked hard to keep him feeling loved and did not point out her absence, as his knowledge of it and the severity of her illness would have caused a great deal of distress for him. When he asked about her, we told him that she was seeing a doctor. He would ask if she was ok, and we would say yes and that she would be home soon. When one episode was life or death, as surgery on a 91-year-old was risky, we took Dad to see her. We believed it was important for Dad and Mom to see each other prior to the surgery despite his likely feeling of helplessness and upset. We were determined to keep him reassured and calm when he went home. At no time would we lie to Dad. We would, however, consider how best to share the truth and how much of that truth to share at the time.

Everyone was to be kind to Dad. There is nothing that can be said more effectively without kindness. As the senses of the aging diminish, their emotional feelings increase. This is even more true of those with Alzheimer's, due to their additional memory loss. They may not remember exactly what was said to them, but they **will** remember how it made them feel. Kindness counts!

Some days, things did not go as planned because something physical, environmental, or emotional caused Dad to be less cooperative. Our approach was to simply ensure that Dad would be safe if we left the room for a few minutes to let him regroup. Then we would walk back in the room and start over, as though nothing had happened.

I have heard it said that a person with Alzheimer's becomes like a child and should be treated as such. I have heard others take great offense to that. In my opinion, the context of the statement determines whether the answer is yes or no. Obviously there are significant differences between a child and an adult. People are patient with children because they are learning. We accept their constant questioning because they do not know and have not known before. They are being taught. An adult living with Alzheimer's has already learned and is forgetting, and yet the people around them find it hard to be patient. When a person living with Alzheimer's has to be retaught a basic skill, they need exactly what a child learning it for the first time needs -- patience. Similarly, when it comes to learning acceptable behavior, children are learning acceptable behavior and the adults with Alzheimer's are trying to remember it. There is a difference however. A child who is learning not to do dangerous things may most effectively be told "No!" The behavior of an adult with Alzheimer's is not effectively modified with "No!" as it is not a matter of them learning or remembering what is unwanted behavior. They simply do not know the difference. Redirection, a useful tool for correcting children, is the best option for getting the wanted results with an adult. Because those with Alzheimer's cannot always remember what they have been told, yet do remember how it made them feel, negative approaches are not helpful and are often hurtful. Adults with Alzheimer's are not children; they remain adults emotionally, yet some of the techniques that are successful with children in learning situations are helpful. Just as children should not be treated as adults, adults should never be treated as though they are children.

Connection

I am often asked what made the biggest difference in the quality of my dad's life. Simply put: basic human connection. Relationships are of highest value. Sadly, by the time Dad was diagnosed with Alzheimer's, he had walked most of his friends through their transition, leaving him only with direct family as support. We do not have a large family, but we are mighty and tenacious. The best thing that anyone could do was to visit Dad, and as often as possible. A visit from a grandchild or great-grandchild was invaluable, as was any visit from a dog.

I have heard some say that they either don't know what to say to someone with Alzheimer's or feel that they have nothing to say to them. Connecting with those with Alzheimer's is like feeding them life-force energy. They require it to exist. Regardless of whether you feel that you have anything to say, be ready to **listen**: be ready, alert and waiting. Listening is a valuable form of connecting.

> Most people do not listen with
> the intent to understand;
> they listen with
> the intent to reply.
> Stephen Covey

As we age, our senses are diminished: sight, taste, smell and lastly, hearing. The sense that does not diminish, and in fact can amplify, is touch. If the diminishing of intellect causes you to feel that you don't know what to say, remember that you can still communicate through the senses. Holding a hand can be worth more than thousands of words. As the senses diminish, emotional memory increases. They feel the energy of a caring soul and the absence of another.

Connection does not have to be verbal. It could be listening to music, maybe singing or dancing to it. Connection can be sitting with the person, not occupied by personal electronics, and watching a movie or sport. We had a caregiver, a young man of 23, who sat patiently holding Dad's hand while they watched a baseball game. The image brings tears to me to this day not only because of the willingness to connect, but also the kindness, compassion and love with which it was done.

Tips That Created Success

First and foremost, we kept Dad's environment as stable as possible: calm, low volume, consistent, positive and loving. We did our best to anticipate what might be distressing to Dad and proactively worked to avoid it. Following is a list of things we did to keep Dad comfortable and at ease, which allowed us to protect his quality of life and reach our goal.

- We were patient and allowed excess time for each task.
  Daily tasks always required more time and rushing was detrimental. When taking Dad out of his home, we allowed for **a lot** of extra time. Rushing was met with resistance, which could escalate into negative behavior.

- We prepared for outings.
  We kept a bag continuously packed with things Dad might need for outings. We also had a list of items to

gather right before an outing that included special supplies, as well as drinks and snacks or meals.

- <u>We played to Dad's strengths.</u>
  We looked for what Dad could do to feel involved and valuable. Whenever our "to do" list included a small but necessary project, such as sealing envelopes or shredding papers, we asked Dad to handle it, sometimes with supervision, so he could take pride in helping us. Dad gave really great back rubs and people requested them. We encouraged Dad to do whatever made him feel valuable.

- <u>We capitalized on cellular memory.</u>
  Certain things are in us as a cellular memory. For many it is music or a skill they have mastered. We played music from the '40s and as soon as we turned the music on, Dad knew every word. Sometimes we would sing, other times we would dance with Dad from his chair. We encouraged playing ball as an exercise and were stunned to see it immediately evoke the basketball skills Dad mastered decades prior. We sat and read or sometimes just looked at the pictures in fishing books, which brought back memories of nearly 80 years of fishing. And we promoted the repetition of everyday skills such as buttoning and using utensils, in order to keep them fresh.

- <u>We continued activities that had always been part of Dad's day.</u>
  o Television Shows
    After a while the current TV shows became overwhelming and distressing. They were too action packed and loud. At first, we found a few British

series that focused more on the characters and story than the action. Dad had more success following British shows, as the speaking was often slower and more distinct. As time went on, we found that old TV shows, ones that Dad had watched many times before, had a familiarity that was comforting.

o Newspapers

Dad was not much of a leisure book reader. His book reading was for learning purposes. Part of his pre-Alzheimer's routine had been to read the newspaper each day. While he had Alzheimer's he would read the newspaper, sometimes several times a day, exercising his reading skills and keeping him feeling part of the world.

o Music

Music is the only activity that activates, stimulates neuroplasticity changes and uses the entire brain. It has proven effects at calming and healing, reducing symptoms of many illnesses and triggering memories and emotions. Many people associate specific events in their lives with specific songs and automatically know the lyrics only when hearing the music. In addition to the benefits of music containing melody and lyrics, orchestral music created a cellular response as Dad had played percussion in his college orchestra. (See *Through the Rabbit Hole* for more detail on the benefits of music.)

- <u>We reinforced his memories.</u>
We had family photos on a digital photo frame, created a large labeled family photo display at the entrance of Dad's bedroom and looked at yearbooks that contained photos of both Dad and Mom.

- We communicated with Dad.

  Whenever we communicated with Dad it was in the context of whatever reality he was experiencing at the time. It didn't have to make sense to us as long as it was not distressful to him.

- We continued to evaluate Dad's needs.

  We constantly considered whether any durable equipment or assistive device would be helpful to Dad. While we used many other devices, such as shower benches and grab bars, the following are specific to either Dad or his living with Alzheimer's.

  o When Dad was in a facility, and because he was tall, we requested an extended length wheelchair and also a raised toilet seat.

  o When we needed the function of a wheelchair, which we had at home, we researched and found a lighter weight transfer chair.

  o When Dad fell out of bed and split his head open on the nightstand, we purchased a quarter length bed rail, not to keep him in bed but rather to prevent his head from hitting the nightstand if he again fell out of bed.

  o As time went on, we found the need for a door alarm so that we would know when Dad had exited his bedroom during the night.

  o As his balance declined we added a motion detector to alert us when he was out of bed. We did not use a bed pad alarm because Dad would often sit up on the side of the bed at night, which would have unnecessarily set off the alarm.

  o Later when he needed assistance in the bathroom, he was extremely sensitive to the coldness of the wipes that we used. A caregiver suggested that we put the adult wipes in a baby wipe warmer, which solved the discomfort agitation.

There are dozens if not hundreds of examples of problems we solved, easily and simply, to improve Dad's comfort and safety. See *Through the Rabbit Hole* for more detail on durable equipment and assistive devices.

🐞🐞 One issue, in regard to Dad's needs, arose unexpectedly when Dad had his first insurance evaluation and was asked if he knew specific things. That approach set him up for failure, and while he was still cognitively capable, he suffered depression afterward when he realized he didn't know certain things. After that, and because he had already been evaluated as qualifying for the insurance, we would not allow such an interview/evaluation again. It was a negative experience for him, one that was unnecessary and detrimental.

- We came up with creative solutions.
  There were constant challenges, some not directly related to living with Alzheimer's but all affecting it.

A problem is a possibility
with a judgement attached to it.
The 2 Bowmans

Following are a couple of examples.
o My dad's bathroom had mirrored walls around the bathtub. He would have to pass the bathtub to reach the toilet. At one point in time, Dad realized that he saw what he thought was his father in the bathroom near the bathtub. It was actually my dad's reflection, which he did not understand, but it was distressing to him even after we explained what was happening.

95

We had to deal with the distress every time he entered the bathroom. My sister's solution was to tape butcher paper over the mirrors in which Dad could see his reflection. Problem solved.

- Television presented some challenges. When Dad's hearing began to deteriorate, we purchased speakers for the TV that allowed the sound to be louder for him without blasting everyone out of the room. We also started putting the subtitles on the TV so that Dad could read them and the volume could be a little lower. The added benefit to the subtitles was that they helped Dad hold on to his reading skills.

- I took Dad to a doctor's appointment and more than an hour later, after having had to provide him with food and take him to the bathroom, the doctor came in. I had spent the entire hour entertaining my dad with everything I could think of. After that, whenever I took Dad to an appointment, my first task after getting Dad settled was to notify someone at the front desk that my dad had Alzheimer's. I politely explained that I understood they were busy but there was a finite window for my dad's compliance, and we would appreciate anything they could do to expedite my dad's appointment. In each and every case, Dad was made a priority and seen very quickly by the doctors.

- Because Dad wanted his clothes always to be clean, we began to need to put something over the top of his shirt when he ate. We did not feel that an adult-sized version of the type of bib worn by young children was a good solution for Dad. Therefore, we purchased decorative cloth napkins and an alligator clip that could be run behind his neck to hold the napkin up over the top of his shirt. It did not look like a bib, nor did he perceive it as such. Of course we always asked permission before placing the alligator clip behind his neck and attaching the napkin.

o I'm not sure if this issue was a direct result of living with Alzheimer's, a result of diminished sight or something else. but Dad began to be a nervous passenger in the car. He would ask "Do you have to go so fast?" when in fact we were going slow. Although nearly the same age, Mom did not have that sensation. The solution was easy, we kept going slow.

- <u>Whenever possible we brought a dog to visit Dad.</u>
He loved them and the benefits of interaction with pets is supported by the visibility of trained pet therapy providers in hospitals and care facilities. Dad would sit with the dog and interact with it, which always calmed him and made him smile. One year a caregiver brought her dog for a visit as a special birthday surprise for Dad. He was delighted.

- <u>Whenever possible grandchildren and great-grandchildren visited.</u>
Visits from Dad's descendants were always the highlight of his day.

- <u>We continued to purchase cards and gifts for Dad to give to Mom.</u>
Dad adored Mom and would have been mortified to think that he had missed recognizing and celebrating an important occasion or holiday. In the early days of Alzheimer's, Dad would fret about not having gotten a card or gift and we would have to constantly assure him that it was handled. Initially we could take Dad to the store to pick out a card and sometimes flowers. When

he could no longer make the trip or the decision, because it was a complex process, we would purchase cards and gifts for him, taking the time to show them to Dad, reading the card if necessary and assisting him to sign his name to the best of his ability. Later in the disease, Mom would tell us not to bother, that it didn't matter to her that he could not do it. But my sisters and I continued to do it, knowing that it was important to Dad.

We also found the following to be effective; again some were not directly related to living with Alzheimer's, but all affected it.

- 2-4 Tablespoons of Coconut oil: When used, we immediately saw improved cognition. Dr. Mary Newport used coconut with her husband who had Alzheimer's and has videos online about her experience. (Google "Dr. Mary Newport" on YouTube.)
- Vitamin D: Dad had spent much of his life outdoors: fishing, playing tennis and skiing. Suddenly his life was nearly completely indoors and his source of vitamin D depleted, contributing to low mood and depression.
- Probiotics: We gave Dad high quality (10 billion organisms) probiotics to assist with his digestion and to boost his immune system. It was especially critical to counter the loss of good bacteria caused by the use of antibiotics.
- D-Mannose: This was helpful in the prevention of urinary tract infections which are prevalent in the elderly. UTIs also cause atypical symptoms at that age.
- Antidepressant: When depression became an issue, we used as low of a dose as possible. The biggest challenge was to figure out the exact time of day to give it to him for optimal benefit.

- <u>Alternative treatments</u>: We maximized what the conventional medical world had to offer Dad for support. In some cases, the conventional treatment was more detrimental than helpful and was discontinued. And we had several unresolved issues that conventional medicine could not address. At one point, after Dad had cried for nearly 38 hours straight, I recall saying that I was open to any alternative method as long as it was noninvasive and didn't involve sticking little pins in little dolls. We did try some unconventional treatments. In every case, the treatment did not require that the participant understand or believe in the technique to obtain positive results. The treatments we chose were successful for Dad. As opposed to listing specific treatment, I would recommend that you do your own research and be open to any legitimate practice. Naturopaths are doctors of naturopathy and offer many holistic and natural options.

Through the Rabbit Hole is a complete resource for successful caregiving.

Having His Ducks in a Row

One of the most important things that my mom ensured was that Dad's estate planning had been completed prior to being diagnosed with Alzheimer's. It is critical that estate planning, including an Advance Directive and final wishes, be created and completed as early in life as possible for everyone. Throughout one's life that planning can be changed as long as the person is deemed competent. A diagnosis of Alzheimer's, or any dementia, starts the clock ticking on how long those changes will be allowed.

At one point, Mom decided to make her power of attorneys concurrent as opposed to consecutive. We were able to have Mom's legal documents changed but could not do the same for Dad because he was unable to legally sign the documents.

Having Dad's estate planning in order made my family's efforts to execute his wishes easier. It was a great gift to have been given.

🐞🐞🐞 Recently I came across a website that now offers an Advance Directive for Dementia, in case one is diagnosed with it. It can be downloaded from www.dementia-directive.org.

Peaceful Endings addresses estate planning in detail.

Sharing the Diagnosis

As I said earlier, Mom decided to tell only her sister and me and my sisters. Virtually no one else knew that Dad had Alzheimer's. Although Mom was a fiercely private woman, I feel that some of that decision was due to the dark stigma that exists. She was correct that any negative projection could be detrimental to Dad.

As we continue to get better at treating Alzheimer's, extending the duration of quality of life and moving closer to prevention and cure, sharing the news with others may be appropriate and even helpful. Dr. Gayatri Devi, in her book, *The Spectrum of Hope*, dedicates a chapter to discussing "When and How to Share the Diagnosis." There are many considerations, specific to the individual diagnosis, which are best discussed in her book. This topic is also covered in *Through the Rabbit Hole*.

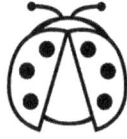

To live in the hearts we leave behind
is not to die.
Ellen G

Chapter 12

HIS LEGACY ...

meaningful beyond the end

> You have no idea what your legacy will be.
> Your legacy is what you do every day.
> Your legacy is every life you've touched,
> every person whose life was either moved or not.
> It's every person you've harmed or helped,
> that's your legacy.
> Maya Angelou

While my experience was more challenging than all the other prior challenges in my life collectively, it was one of the most rewarding experiences and opportunities of my life.

> They say that what doesn't kill you
> makes you stronger, at this point,
> I should be able to bench-press a Buick.
> Unknown

While it was filled with challenges, it was also filled with humor, precious moments that occurred spontaneously and made us feel lucky to witness, and more love than I can describe.

In our country, Alzheimer's is often thought of as a death sentence. People are treated as though they are stupid, which only shows our ignorance. After all, it is not their intelligence that is affected but their memory and ability to organize complex thoughts. They still have a lot – memories (mental image, smell); a sense of humor; a sense of knowing (tribe/clan); the ability to have a quality, meaningful life; and the capacity to love.

I learned more in 21 months than I did in the 54 years before that. And my classroom was primarily a small family room, 10 ft. x 10 ft. It was an inclusive environment where everyone who entered was part of Dad's tribe, his trusted clan. If they got past the front door, he knew that they were "safe." Dad and Alzheimer's brought wonderful people to us, people who have not only affected, but who will hopefully be in our lives forever. Dad always said that family is everything, and in addition to bringing our family closer together, he brought us a new family of caregivers.

> Diamonds are carbon
> under a lot of heat and pressure.
> Trish Laub

Alzheimer's presented physical demands and mental challenges and required emotional stamina at previously incomprehensible levels, and required me to do things that I could never have imagined. I learned that I am stronger than I could ever have dreamed; love allows you to go way beyond anything you ever thought possible. And, that in the midst of overwhelming stress, critical and ongoing traumas, there is invaluable knowledge and unforeseen treasures.

It takes selflessness to give time back to our parents, as they gave us time when we were young. I understand that not everyone has a positive relationship with their parents, and that in some cases bad things happened. Regardless, it is not about the past; it is about the present moment and the future. It's about doing what is feasible and what is right, and about what will make life ok for you in the future. It calls into question selfishness, excuses, integrity, and right and wrong, causing you to evaluate what life is about and of what you as a human being are made. It is the opportunity of a lifetime to re-evaluate what you stand for and what you believe. And it will impact every relationship in your life. It will show you who your spouse is, who your siblings are, and who your real friends are. You will learn who rationalizes their excuses and who shows up to do the hard work.

> How you treat someone else
> says more about you,
> than it does about them.
> Trish Laub

I learned to make decisions, sometimes life and death, on the fly often on no sleep and without enough information to make a well-analyzed decision; to rely on my gut, my 6th sense, not thinking but instead knowing what the right answer was, often factoring dozens of aspects and evaluating them seemingly on auto pilot from outside the situation. When you put the best interest of the other person first, the answers are easy. In the end, a dear old friend, who had watched our care situation unfold, said that I appeared "undaunted."

> We're reflections of the people
> who have loved us selflessly.
> Bob Goff

While I never wanted to lose my dad, I wanted more for him not to struggle or suffer. I had been told that death from Alzheimer's could be awful, but anything, including longevity, that causes the body to shut down is most likely unpleasant. So my hope always was that my dad would pass away before things got unpleasant for him. I wanted more for him than I wanted for myself. As the time of his passing neared, all material possessions and his identity based on accomplishments fell away one by one, until my dad lay in his bed, in his own home surrounded by those who loved him most, and quietly and peacefully slipped into pure light. With the grace of hospice, his death process was not awful but instead painless and peaceful, and most importantly, on his terms.

My great nephew Will said it best, "He's always so sad when you leave because he loves you so much." In the final days and hours of life, all the things that many think are important and allow to occupy their time, drift away and it all comes down to one thing – love.

> Life is a series of pulls back and forth …
> a tension of opposites,
> like the pull on a rubber band.
> And most of us live somewhere in the middle.
> Which side wins? Love always wins.
> Morrie Schwartz from *Tuesdays with Morrie*

What was my dad's legacy? With all of his credentials, his greatest accomplishment was his role as husband and father. He was one of the two most truly decent humans I will ever know. The other is my mom, Dad's reason to succeed and his anchor to reality till the end. Dad's legacy: simply, love. He had a heart, so pure and strong, that loved completely: his family, his friends, our friends, those who needed his care, and in the end, those who cared for him. He was a hero to many, and a champion for others, as he truly cared to make a difference for each person if only by listening, providing a hand up, or encouraging them to be their best. Even in his final days, he helped women to heal and inspired boys to become men. He touched the lives of many, which were never the same.

We all need someone
who inspires us to do better
than we know how.
Unknown

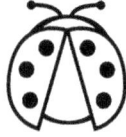

No one is useless in this world
who lightens the burdens of another.
Charles Dickens

Chapter 13

TESTAMENTS TO A MOST MEANINGFUL LIFE ...
in others' words

It was Margery, a caregiver, who suggested that I write about our collective experience with my dad and Alzheimer's. She also suggested that I request that our caregivers write something, anything, about the time they spent with Dad, and she came up with the name *A Most Meaningful Life*. For that I will always be grateful. The letter that Margery wrote is the Introduction to this book. Below are some of those letters and a couple of the hundreds of condolences we received. They are a testament to the fact that Dad lived a most meaningful life, with Alzheimer's, through his final days.

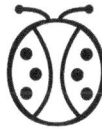

Frank will live on in the hearts and minds of those he has touched and positively influenced over the years and his good deeds. **I am thankful for the ways in which he has touched my life** and some of the fun fishing experiences shared, and his FBI "stories" embellished on a bit I am sure. Frank was a man's man and will live on forever in the memorable experiences we all shared with him.

Jim, family friend

Frank was one of the coolest guys I've met. I only had the privilege of knowing him for about eight months of his positive accomplished life, and in those eight months not only did I learn who Frank was through short stories he told me, but **he also motivated me to be what I can be in life.**

At the age of 91, Frank had great skills with his little ball. There were nights we sat there and played ball, talked all night, or nights Mr. Frank slept all night.

Coming to work I never knew what to expect, but every time I left his house that's all my family talked about. He was like part of our family through the different stories I shared with my family. Frank will be greatly missed.

Shawn, caregiver

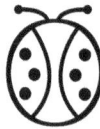

He was always smiling, always in a good mood, always serene. Frank was always happy to see me. I knew I was safe with Frank. **He would always have a kind word for me, and I basked in his kindness.**

What a legacy your father has left all of you: **to have so many talents but to put his most valuable energy into loving you.**

He died knowing that you loved him and you live knowing that he loved you. That is beautiful and the love will last forever.

Excerpts from Nonnie, family friend

Frank was a most kind and gentle man. He reminded me daily of my dad.

In watching Frank, you could see that he had such life in his eyes and his speech when responding to the love of his life, his wife, Jean. He showed such tenderness with his touch.

Seeing Frank and Jean together whether they were talking, not talking, or just looking at each other was truly like a fairy tale.

You could tell what a great Dad he was to his daughters. His face would always light up. He joked, played and responded to each of them. Such love he had for each one. What a pleasure to see a parent and children love each other the way you do.

Frank took such good pride in how he looked and dressed. He had such a great sense of humor, loved to sing and direct. Loved to play ball, tell jokes with a twinkle in his eyes.

Ah, sweets he loved – Frank had such a love of food, especially desserts.

I loved to see Frank play ball with family members; he always laughed – such a laugh he would have.

Frank had such a love for family and life. I am honored to have known and been able to have taken care of him. He shall be missed greatly.

Much love to his wife Jean and his daughters – my extended family.

Lucia, caregiver

I was awarded a very great opportunity and offered a spot on a great team, and in doing so, I was given the great pleasure to take care of Frank. As a caregiver, I would talk with Frank, watch over him and provide help. Frank being very independent didn't need much, so the time we spent together consisted of many things from talking, watching TV, grabbing arms and dancing, play shooting and peek-a-boo. In this time Frank and I grew a bond, and **I eventually looked at Frank as a grandpa as opposed to a client**. The time I had with Frank was great and irreplaceable. Taking time to get to know Frank opened doors and I was able to meet Frank's close family including his wife and three daughters. Many stories shared through the family revealed how great of a person Frank actually was. I could have been having a horrible day and go to take care of Frank and the atmosphere that Frank and his family created just changed everything. A smile ear to ear bigger than the Grinch, Frank would greet me as I walked in. Always caring and worried more about others than himself, he was always quick to ask about my day and how I was. While working with Frank, he did get sick a couple of times. Being there the last time seeing Frank sick was hard, horrible, as two of my family members and I knew Frank and his family. My family and I did all we could to keep Frank comfortable. Frank then passed. That was one of the hardest things, it affected Frank's family a lot, and since we see Frank and his family as ours, we were impacted in a major way as well. Seeing Frank as a grandpa I wish I had, I felt I lost a best friend. Now that he was in a better place, we were able to celebrate Frank's life, which did help me get past that point. Rest in Paradise Frank, you are missed….

David, caregiver

To me, I feel Frank was a very caring person. If Mr. Frank thought he was being difficult he would apologize.

Frank gave the best massages ever; he was so content when he would be doing it. Mr. Frank loved looking at pictures of his family. He would tell me things about the pictures and would have a great big smile and did he ever have a great smile. I loved when I would get him up in the morning and he would have **that great contagious smile**. I will miss that when I think of him and that smile, I also smile with a little sadness. I feel very lucky to have been able to care for such a caring and lovely man.

Debbie, caregiver

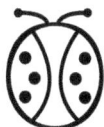

I will always remember **how welcome Jean and Frank made me feel** whenever I visited your River Forest home, and I can still hear his jovial voice greeting me.

Roseanne, family friend

Frank has a way of making you feel at ease and making you comfortable, which helped when you were shy or first nervous about starting a new job.

Frank loved to be silly and joke around which helped you get in touch with your inner child and just relax and let the day's stress go away.

Frank would always give you a compliment which in turn would boost your confidence and truly make you feel better.

Frank did all these things with everyone he met. Frank made you want to be a better person, he made you feel like you were part of the family, and I looked at Frank as a grandfather always there, always smiling, always making you feel better.

Frank is truly a one-of-a-kind gentleman, and I feel **he has made me a better person** just by knowing him.

Angel, caregiver

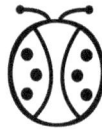

I will treasure my memories of this sweet gentleman from The Greatest Generation, who was, as you know, like my second dad - such a central figure in my childhood. He lived a full, happy life and **his loving family is but one of his lasting tributes**.

Jennifer, family friend

Papa Frank

I lost my father in 2005, and till today it seems like yesterday. It never passes a day before I remember him. My father had a lot of similarities to Frank; he was kind, loving, caring, respectful and funny. **I used to call Frank Papa, to me he was my papa too and I called him Papa with all the respect it carried, and I meant it.** I loved and respected him as if he was my own father. I miss him dearly, and I remember him all the time. Whenever I would come to work after his passing, I would look at his chair, his stool and I would miss him too much and my heart would feel cold.

My day with papa Frank used to start either from the bathroom or his bedroom. I would go greet him, then I would dance for him; sometimes he would be so excited, he would laugh or clap. I would tell him after the dance it was nice to see him, and he would tell me it was nice to see me too. That would make my day! During the dance he would say "wow, look at her." Another time he said, "oh man; she is wild." I remember this day I found him sitting on his bed, not long before he passed, but for some reason he was in a very good mood. I held his hand, and I started singing for him "you are my sunshine, my only sunshine." He joined me and together we sang the whole song, it was beautiful! I have never seen him smile that big!

One morning I came when it was snowing, I told him I was afraid of driving in the snow, and where I came from it never snows. He reached out for my hand and he told me, "don't worry I will help you." Frank was caring that much. Another night I was going home, and after I said goodnight to him he told me "Thank you, I am at peace." Not long before this he fell sick. As he said, yes he is at peace now, no more pain, no more suffering.

Papa Frank was a very loving person, many times he would look at Ms. Jean and he would call to her "mummy is everything ok, are you ok?" At times one could not help to see his frustration and helplessness; he was feeling he needed to help his wife more but he could not. He would start crying at times and he would say, "I can't do anything." But Ms. Jean with her calm peaceful voice would tell him "Hi love, I am ok, and the girls are ok, too. They will be coming soon to visit us" and he would say "Is it?" then he would sit back in his chair and sleep.

Another time as I was playing ball with him, he told me I had been there for a long time and he asked me when I go home. I told him soon, and he told me "I will pay you overtime." That shows Frank was a loving caring person, and I loved and appreciated him for that.

I will never forget soon before he passed on Nancy and I were taking care of him, and Nancy told him "Dad I am here with my Kenyan friend." After we were done, Papa Frank said "thank you both of you." Despite the pain and discomfort, he was going through during those last days, he never forgot to say "thank you," "I love you," "I am sorry."

I cannot forget this one day he got mad with me for taking away his plate without his permission, he told me "go jump in the sea." I told him "but I don't know how to swim." Then you drown, he said. It was funny the way he said it. But anytime Papa would tell you something that was not pleasant, it used to make him feel so bad. Soon he would look at you and say "I am sorry, you are a good girl."

All we can say Papa is:

May the road rise up to meet you,
May the wind be always at your back,
May the sun shine warm upon your face,
May rains fall soft upon your fields,
And until we meet again,
May God hold you in the palm of His hand.
Traditional Irish Prayer.

Ann, caregiver

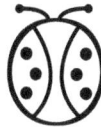

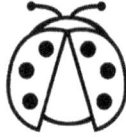

Alzheimer's is a new stage
in a wonderful life,
no less challenging
or interesting
than all the earlier stages.
Cathleen McBride, diagnosed with Alzheimer's,
from *The Spectrum of Hope*

Chapter 14

FINAL THOUGHTS ...
and additional reading

Alzheimer's is a marathon, not a sprint. My daughter who runs marathons says that how you recover is based on how you prepared. If you did your training according to the time-tested schedule for runs, you will recover from the full event more quickly. If not, you will suffer. Similarly, how you plan for caregiving will determine whether you survive or thrive during the experience.

As I said in the beginning, this book is specific to Alzheimer's, but there is much information that is needed that is not disease specific: estate planning, dignified caregiving and end of life.

The philosophy, goal and strategy may be different for every person. What is important is that you identify them before you are hit with a crisis. Part of the process is to talk to your loved ones or those whose care you may oversee. Make your wishes known, through estate planning and documentation, and then learn the wishes of your family members. Know what the goal is and what the strategy might be: in-home or facility care, based on the insurance and financial options. Start to create a plan, because the day you hear the diagnosis is not the time to start planning. Yes, Alzheimer's usually offers many stages, so there will be time to clarify and detail your plan, but at least the necessary discussions and thought processes will have begun. The more those you love are prepared with estate planning, and the more you are prepared (truly the greatest gift you can give your loved ones), the more life can go on as usual for as long as possible.

You need to have a plan, the basic structure or outline, which can be modified over time.

Throughout my experience, and in part because of the projected statistics on Alzheimer's and other dementias, what became obvious to me is that we have a responsibility as a society to be prepared, to educate ourselves in order to do better, and to do the best that we can to both prevent dementia and prepare to provide care for those with it. The statistics don't say if, but rather when, we will have to deal with it. I didn't see Alzheimer's coming and certainly wasn't prepared. I truly wish I had been.

I am already one of the Alzheimer's statistics, having been a caregiver for a family member. I don't know if I will have the disease, or if I will care for another with it. But I do know that I have choices.

1. I choose to be <u>optimistic</u> about the future.
We live in a time when medical advances and research happen at warp speed. There is much about which to be optimistic:
- New thoughts on causes and possible prevention
- New medications on the horizon
- New approaches and techniques
    - Ultrasound to break up plaque
    - Transcranial Magnetic Stimulation (TMS) to improve language, motor, and life skills
    - EVOX for emotional reframing of distressful emotional memories
- New thoughts on Alzheimer's as a spectrum disease
- Research continues: For example, in October 2017, Bill Gates donated $50 million of his personal money to work toward finding a cure for Alzheimer's.

and

2. I choose to be <u>kind</u>. My experience with Alzheimer's tells me that the disease has great potential to amplify a person's natural tendencies. Therefore, I choose to be kind so that if I eventually live with Alzheimer's, I will be kind to those who help me to remain independent and who later care for me.

Following is a list of some of the topics covered in *Through the Rabbit Hole* and *Peaceful Endings* that serve as a supplement to the information in *A Most Meaningful Life* and guide the way through estate planning, dignified caregiving and end of life.

Through the Rabbit Hole details the following and more:
- Crisis management
- A new responsibility
- Care options and approaches
- Worthwhile assistive items and durable equipment
- Dealing with specific medical issues

Peaceful Endings details the following and more:
- Crisis management
- Getting started
- Understanding estate planning
- Palliative and hospice care
- The final stretch
- After transition
- Settling an estate
- Moving forward
- Pre-emptive preparedness

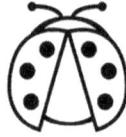

I'm a strong person
but every once in a while,
I would like someone to take my hand
and tell me
that everything's going to be all right.
Unknown

POSTSCRIPT ...

The first thing to understand is that a person in crisis needs help. They may not be able to ask for it. Sometimes they are too exhausted to know what they need or to even make the effort to ask for help. Everyone in a tough situation can use support. There is helpful support and misguided support. Knowing the difference makes all the difference to the one in need.

Move Love Inward, Throw The "Trash" Outward

Often at the height of a crisis, people find that they not only feel they don't know what is appropriate or helpful to say but that they in fact have said the wrong thing unintentionally.

For decades I have been aware of my relationships with others, even distinguishing between real friends and acquaintances, where real friends are let into an imaginary circle allowing them to be closer to me than acquaintances who reside in a circle further away from me. *Susan Silk, a clinical psychologist, and Barry Goldman describe a way to use that imagery to help identity what is and is not appropriate and helpful for others to say to someone in a crisis situation.* They suggest the following, which I have enhanced.

Draw a circle and write the name of the person in crisis in the center.

Draw six more circles, each larger and outside of the previous.

Label the circles, starting with the circle closest to the original, as follows

circle #2:	immediate family: significant other, children
circle #3:	close family: parents, siblings
circle #4:	true friends
circle #5:	colleagues
circle #6:	acquaintances, distant relatives
circle #7:	anyone else

The rule is simple: send your *love inward* and your *"trash" outward*.

The person in the center can say anything, positive or negative, to anyone at any time.

For every other circle, the intention is to help those closer to the crisis, those in the smaller circles. Therefore, listening is more helpful than talking, which should provide only comfort and support. Advice should not be given to those in a smaller circle, only love and support get put in. "Trash", complaining or unhelpful personal experience or information, should be shared with bigger circles only. The trash should always be dumped out.

Most people know not to dump trash into the center ring, but many don't realize that it is never helpful to dump into any smaller circle.

Susan Silk is a clinical psychologist. Barry Goldman is an arbitrator and mediator and the author of "The Science of Settlement: Ideas for Negotiators."
OpEd piece in the LA Times 2007
http://articles.latimes.com/2013/apr/07/opinion/la-oe-0407-silk-ring-theory-20130407

What You Can Do to Help Someone in Crisis

The needs of people are variable during a time of crisis. The intensity of the crisis will ebb and flow, and with it the needs. Some crises are a sprint to a cure or a premature end and others a marathon of treatment and care. Every situation is different depending on whether the person is at home or in a facility, there are caregivers and which type, how long the crisis is likely to last and what will happen once the crisis is resolved. The person in crisis may be the caregiver (spouse, family member, friend) and/or the person needing care.

Some people will be able to provide emotional support, others logistical support and others will be organizers. If everyone uses their strengths to provide help, the person in crisis will be lifted up as much as possible.

First, ask…. "How can I help?" If you get an answer, do it. If you do not get an answer, make a suggestion, such as asking if receiving a dinner would be helpful. Sometimes people are not comfortable with accepting help, let alone asking for it. It is optimal if the person can articulate their needs. If not, sometimes it is easier for them to acknowledge whether or not a specific offer would be helpful at that time, and the offer allows them to suggest something different such as lunch instead of dinner. If you hear hesitance in their voice, you can always drop something off at their home and make it clear that you do not expect to stay and visit. If they are in need of a visit, they will invite you.

Gift cards to restaurants, in particular those offering carry out, are thoughtful. Sometimes having a gift card is the difference between whether or not the person stops to get food.

If the crisis is ongoing, you can offer to set up a calendar of food/meal deliveries, errands to be run, housecleaning etc. Ask for a list of people to contact.

Respite for the caregiver comes in many forms. If appropriate, something to brighten the person's day is nice. Think in terms of something they particularly enjoy: flowers, a sweet treat, a message, a book, or anything that will provide a moment's respite from the stress. Respite might include a visit with the person in crisis, allowing an intellectual and emotional respite for the caregiver, as well as the person being cared for, by changing the focus for a brief time. If the situation requires full-time care, a longer visit can provide the caregiver time to recharge and rejuvenate.

Whatever the method, support from friends is often what keeps someone dealing with a crisis afloat. Something as simple as a message saying that you are thinking about them can make all the difference in their day. And never underestimate the power of just listening or lending a shoulder on which to cry.

OTHER RESOURCES

Listed are few of the resources that I found most helpful. Visit www.TrishLaub.com for more resources.

The Comfort in Their Journey Book Series by Trish Laub
A Most Meaningful Life
        my dad and Alzheimer's
Peaceful Endings
        guiding the walk to the end of life and beyond
Through the Rabbit Hole
        navigating the maze of providing care

Alzheimer's
Alzheimer's Association
www.Alz.org
The Alzheimer's Association is an invaluable resource for anyone affected by Alzheimer's. Provides family consultation and support groups, classes, a 24-hour bilingual helpline, and safety programs that are available free of charge through individual state chapters.

Be with me Today
        A challenge to the Alzheimer's outside
By Richard Taylor, Ph.D.
DVD: HaveAGoodLife.com
A psychologist and professor diagnosed with Alzheimer's at 58 explains what it is like to have the disease, how people treat him and how they should treat him – that there is a person in there.

Contented Dementia
By Oliver James
Based on the SPECAL (Specialized Early Care for Alzheimer's) method, this book delves into the feelings and past memories that remain intact in a person living with Alzheimer's, and how both can be used to create links to the loss of more recent information.

Gates Notes, the blog of Bill Gates   www.gatesnotes.com
Why I'm digging deep into Alzheimer's blogpost

I'm Still Here
        A New Philosophy of Alzheimer's Care
By John Zeisel, Ph.D.
I'm Still Here is a guidebook to Dr. Zeisel's treatment ideas, showing the possibility and benefits of connecting with an Alzheimer's patient through their abilities that don't diminish with time, thereby offering a quality of life with connection to others.

The Spectrum of Hope,
        An Optimistic and New Approach to Alzheimer's
        Disease and Other Dementias
By Gayatri Devi, M.D.
The author defines Alzheimer's as a spectrum disease that affects different people differently. She encourages early treatment which enables doctors and caregivers to effectively manage the disease, allowing those diagnosed with it to continue to live fulfilling lives.

Dignified Care

Being Mortal
Medicine and What Matters in the End
By Atul Gawande
In the inevitable condition of aging and death, the goals of medicine too frequently run counter to the interest of the human spirit. This book offers examples of freer, more socially fulfilling models for assisting the aging and end of life.

Honest Medicine
Shattering the myths about aging and health care
By Donald J Dr. Murphy, M.D.
Dr. Murphy sets the record straight on popular myths, mistakes and misconceptions in regard to the controversial issues associated with health care for older patients and the importance of understanding the pros and cons of treatments.

Learning from Hannah
Secrets for a Life Worth Living
By William H. Thomas, M.D.
Through storytelling, this book addresses the value of elders to the community as a whole and focuses on 10 principles necessary to meet their needs which include eliminating the three greatest causes of suffering: loneliness, helplessness and boredom. The 10 principles have become the basis for a real-world project, the Eden Alternative, dedicated to creating quality of life for elders and their care partners, wherever they may live.

Life After the Diagnosis
    Expert Advice on Living Well with Serious Illness
    for Patients and Caregivers
By Steven Z. Pantilat, MD
A guide to living well with serious illness and getting the best possible end-of-life care.

End of Life

The Life Changing Magic of Tidying Up
> The Japanese art of decluttering and organizing

By Marie Kondo
This book offers a strategy for sorting through volumes of items, identifying what r what to pass along.

When Breath Becomes Air
By Paul Kalanithi
A neurosurgeon's perspective as a patient with stage 4 lung cancer and the question of what makes a life worth living.

When Souls Take Flight
> coping with grief

By Kira Rosner
A non-sectarian view of what happens when we die, with compassionate advice for anyone who is grieving.

ABOUT THE AUTHOR

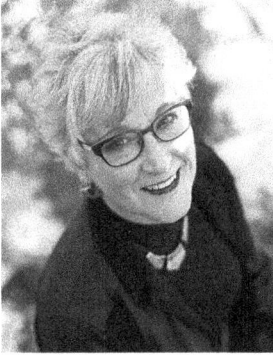

In 2002 Trish Laub was told that her father was being treated for Alzheimer's. Originally from Chicago, she and her husband moved to the Denver area in 2012 not only to enjoy the beautiful mountains but also to be closer to her parents.

Just 48 hours after Trish arrived in town, her father experienced an unexpected medical crisis, setting into motion a two and one-half year journey of care. Trish served as not only a caregiver but also as manager of both the care team and her parents' medical care. The process continued through their end of life and the settlement of their estate, and has since included the care of her mother-in-law and consulting for others. In all, over a period of five years, Trish has gained over 12,000 hours of experience in providing care for a loved one, including one living with Alzheimer's, taking the final walk of their life with them, and settling their estates.

After spending 18 years developing computer systems, Trish went on to co-found both a national dance education company and a national nonprofit prevention theater company focused on helping at-risk teens. She is a Black Belt instructor of The Nia Technique and has been licensed since 1999. Using her previous computer and teaching experience in combination with her most recent caregiving experience, Trish has created Comfort in Their Journey to provide practical guidance for dignified care through end of life.

134

Trish Laub
Author | Consultant | Speaker

AUTHOR

Trish is available to present her book series to your audience and to offer signed copies.

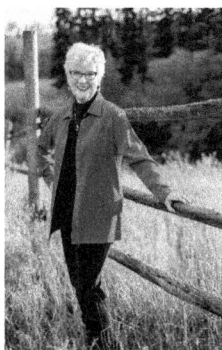

SPEAKER

Schedule Trish to bring her expertise to your group. Trish offers a variety of presentations on Alzheimer's, crisis management, end-of-life and dignified care, or can create a custom presentation for your group. She presents concise and specific information that is immediately useful, and inspires her audiences with the goal of teaching others to provide compassionate and dignified care.

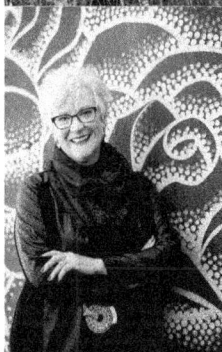

CONSULTANT

Consult Trish for guidance on meeting your caregiving needs. Trish is available to help you address your caregiving needs by discussing care options and answering your questions.

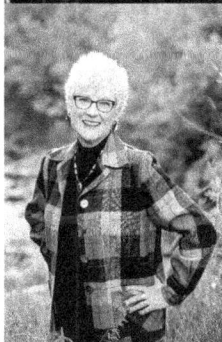

www.TrishLaub.com
720-288-0772

THE COMFORT IN THEIR JOURNEY
BOOK SERIES

A Most Meaningful Life
my dad and Alzheimer's
a guide to living with dementia

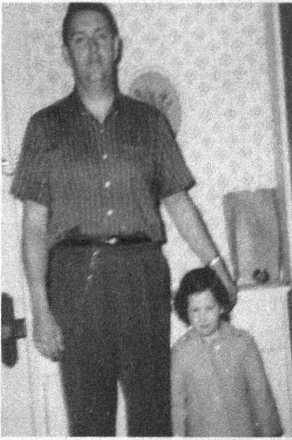

A Most Meaningful Life
my dad and Alzheimer's

a guide to living with dementia
Trish Laub

A Most Meaningful Life tells the story of a daughter's journey through Alzheimer's disease with her father, from her initial awareness of his diagnosis to navigating his care and helping him achieve the good death that we all deserve. It is the story of how Alzheimer's affected her father's life and the lives of those who loved him, as well as the story of her family's successes and failures throughout the journey. With her family's efforts, creativity and desire to preserve their father's quality of life for over a decade, he continued to truly live a meaningful life through his final days.

Through the story of her journey, the author offers a new perspective, the determination that even with Alzheimer's, the possibilities are limitless. With a clear philosophy and the creation of a strategy, others can have a roadmap to navigate their loved one's journey so that they have "A Most Meaningful Life."

Peaceful Endings
guiding the walk to the end of life and beyond
steps to take before and after

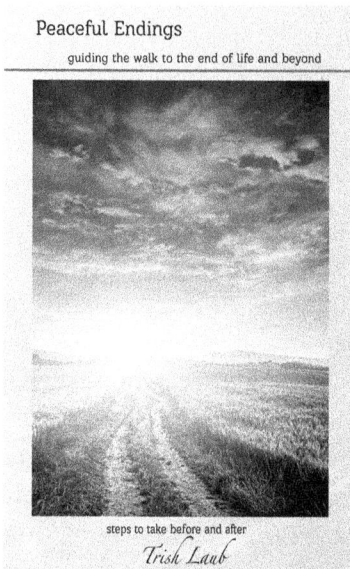

Peaceful Endings
guiding the walk to the end of life and beyond

steps to take before and after
Trish Laub

The topic "no one wants to talk about," end of life and beyond, is exactly what *Peaceful Endings* addresses. Many times the end of life is preceded by illness and caregiving, and may also include a variety of crises, as life changes and decisions must be made quickly. Whether proactively preparing for the end of life, or facing it imminently, there are medical, legal, financial, insurance and care decisions to be made, each with its own specific language. The author walks the reader through the terminology, the choices and the process of the end of life. The author also details what must be done after the transition, and provides perspective on stepping into a new normal after a loved one's life has ended.

Through the Rabbit Hole
navigating the maze of providing care
a quick guide to care options and decisions

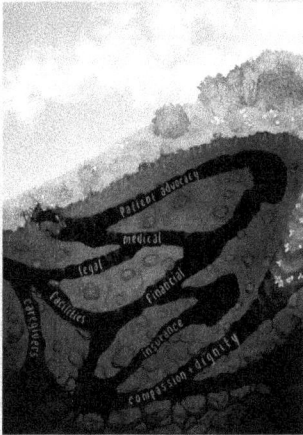

Through the Rabbit Hole

navigating the maze of providing care

a quick guide to care options and decisions

Trish Laub

Through the Rabbit Hole is exactly the reference book that the author needed for quick access to information during her experience providing care for her ill parents. It wasn't available for her, so she has written it for all the families and caregivers who are now beginning their journeys. Her parents' medical crises caused her to fall down the rabbit hole and into the maze of unfamiliar options and decisions. Having emerged from the maze, the author details the complexities of caregivers and facilities, the need for patient advocacy, as well as the medical, legal, financial and insurance aspects of care. With the end goal of compassionate and dignified care, this book, a wonderful companion to *A Most Meaningful Life*, is a beacon through the maze of care.

Comfort in their Journey
with *Trish Laub*

Whether during an illness or injury, or at the end of life, I hope that you have found your purchase helpful in your journey of providing compassionate and dignified care.

VISIT THE COMFORT IN THEIR JOURNEY WEBSITE

Go to www.TrishLaub.com to check out everything Trish has to offer including a blog containing new information and topics not covered in the book series.

While you are there… please send us a review to post.

COMING IN SPRING 2019

The CitJClub membership including access to the information in all three books in the series, including search capabilities across all three books, and much more.

Your purchase of this book qualifies you for a discounted CitJClub membership.
Visit www.TrishLaub.com for more information.
720-288-0772

.

www.ingramcontent.com/pod-product-compliance
Lightning Source LLC
Chambersburg PA
CBHW062108040426
42336CB00042B/2668